THE 60-DAY DIET DIARY

WRITTEN BY KAREN KREPS
WITH DRAWINGS BY
RICHARD SMITH

A DELL TRADE PAPERBACK

PRODUCED BY THE ALEXANDER SMITH COMPANY

A DELL TRADE PAPERBACK

Published by
Dell Publishing
a division of
The Bantam Doubleday Dell Publishing Group, Inc.
666 Fifth Avenue
New York, New York 10103

ISBN: 0-440-57946-5

Printed in the United States of America

Five Previous Editions

January 1987

10

FG

INTRODUCTION

Quick! What did you eat for dinner last night? You *do* remember. Good. But how about the night before? And what did you have for lunch last Wednesday? Did you snack on Saturday afternoon? On what? And how many drinks did you down at the reception the other day? Can't remember? Think it doesn't matter?

You may forget the food you eat, but the calories you consume are not so easily forgotten. Any extra calories that are not expended by your daily activity will be stored as fat. So if you want to know where those extra ten pounds came from, or how you acquired that tire you tote around your midriff, it might be a good idea to take a careful inventory of everything you've been putting into your body. Keeping track of what you eat can tell you how you got out of shape, and more importantly, it is the best way to get back *into* shape.

The 60-Day Diet Diary is a diet book, but it is not a diet. It recommends no particular regimen or method of weight reduction. Rather, it is a nonpartisan support system that can be used as a companion to any diet. You will find it helpful if you're on the Scarsdale, Stillman, Atkins, Weight Watchers, or any other prescribed or improvised diet. In fact, you can use this book even if you aren't on a diet. Use it to monitor your current weight, to keep track of the nutrients you're putting into your body, or to keep tabs on how much money you are spending on food every day. Here's how it works:

The 60-Day Diet Diary will be your friend and dining companion for the next two months. You may begin at any time. Just turn to page 11 and write in the date at the top. Very simply, you should write down *everything* you eat and drink immediately after you consume it. Don't attempt to record the menu at the end of the day; you're bound to forget some of the details. Keep this book in your briefcase or handbag so you can refer to it regularly. Jot down not only your meals but your snacks, between-meal beverages, after-work drinks, and midnight pantry raids. Put it all down. Don't worry, no one but you need see this book; it is your own, very personal diary.

Counting calories is an intellectual activity, but eating is an emotional process. Jot down what your mood was like at the time you ate. Record your feelings with a simple word or two such as *self-confident, bored, angry, nervous, irritable, excited, tired, sad, frustrated, peaceful, cheerful,* or *restless.* It's important for you to get in touch with how you are feeling when you eat. Discover your motivations. You may find that you eat for dozens of reasons that have nothing whatever to do with hunger.

It's also important to write down the time at which you ate, and where or with whom you were. Become aware of danger areas—times of the day in which you ate out of habit. Did you pig-out just because your family decided to make a stop at a dairy stand? Notice if you're eating only to fulfill social conventions, or because you're with someone who is a big eater. Is there a way to avoid those situations?

The other important part of your record-keeping is your daily weigh-in. It's best to weigh yourself first thing in the morning, without clothes, and on the same scale. Record your weight in the blank at the top of that day's page. Water retention can cause your weight to fluctuate as much as two to three pounds from day to day—even when you're sticking faithfully to your diet—so don't be discouraged if you show a weight gain for no apparent reason. Your weight may just as suddenly go down again! What's most important is that you record your weight every day, and getting onto the scale each morning is a good impetus for you to use *The 60-Day Diet Diary* effectively throughout the rest of the day.

You can also chart your weight reduction by keeping track of your body size. In the beginning, middle, and end of *The 60-Day Diet Diary* there are places for you to paste or staple a photograph of yourself and to write in your measurements. Being able to wear your favorite belt a couple of notches tighter can be a great source of inspiration.

Whether you gain, lose, or stabilize your weight depends on how you balance the calories you consume against the calories you burn. A calorie, simply, is a quantity of food capable of producing a certain amount of energy when it is burned in the body's metabolic system. Any that are not burned are stored as fat.

Pages 134–144 of *The 60-Day Diary* contain an extensive listing of the caloric values of most of the foods you are likely to eat. Obviously, you won't always be able to scale your portions to the amounts listed. The important thing is to be aware of what you eat, how many calories each food contains, and how they can add up in a day's time. Another thing to remember when you read the dieting tips in this book that describe how many calories are burned in a particular activity like swimming or dancing is that a large-sized person burns more calories doing an activity than a small-sized person doing the same thing. For example, if a 170-pound man and a 110-pound woman take an hour-long walk together, the man will burn 372 calories while the woman will burn only 270 calories. The numbers of calories listed as being burned in the various tips generally refer to a 140-pound person.

More and more people are making physical exercise an important part of their daily health routine. While it takes a great deal of intensive exercise to actually burn off fat, a regular program of moderate exercise will help you tone and recondition droopy muscles and tighten skin that has been stretched by excess weight. And a well-toned body not only looks better, it feels better! We leave it to you to choose an exercise regimen from one of the many that are available in books or formal classes at health clubs, YMCAs, etc. But once you've chosen your exercise program, your goal becomes the same as for your diet: to do it every day and record your activity in the space provided on the right-hand pages of *The 60-Day Diet Diary.*

Don't be afraid to write down the times you skipped the exercise or went off your diet. Don't make dieting an all-or-nothing proposition. We all slip up; it's only human. Right now, make a commitment to stick to your diet plans at least until all the pages of this book are filled. If along the way you stumble, it's no reason to stop. Let your follies inspire you to indulge in a little more activity the next day, or to cut out more calories—or both. Dieting is a means, not an end. Every little effort and attempt that you make has a cumulative effect. It makes you stronger and brings you closer to your goal.

If you want to see daily progress, set up sub-goals that have to do with exercising self-control. Acknowledge the victory when you manage to spend an entire week eating only healthy foods. Write down for posterity that you successfully resisted taking a second helping of dessert. It is equally important to acknowledge your triumphs as well as your failures.

The buddy system is a great source of inspiration. Find a friend to be your diet buddy. (Someone from work is ideal because you see him or her regularly, and it will help build a sense of trust and a relationship between you and your co-worker.) Give him or her a copy of *The 60-Day Diet Diary* and compare notes. Report to each other every day on your progress, and make a pact that you may call each other at any hour of the day or night rather than raid the refrigerator.

But you'll find the best source of inspiration written in your own handwriting on the right-hand pages of this book. Take a look at all the food that you've consumed in a week. Picture it all together, think about its weight and quantity, and then, mentally try to squeeze all that food and drink into your body. It doesn't fit? Good. You don't need to add anything more to the list. Every time you're about to eat something, think, How will this look in *The 60-Day Diet Diary?*

Once the sixty days have passed, don't discard this book. Keep it around and it will continue to serve as a source of inspiration. Should you begin to regain weight, look over your entries to see if your eating habits have reverted into an old, unhealthy pattern. The very act of recalling the diet process may put you back on the right track.

Okay, it's time to begin. Nervous because you never before were the hero of a book? Well, don't hesitate. Just remember, you have nothing to gain by using this book. YOU HAVE EVERYTHING TO LOSE.

FULL LENGTH PHOTO
DAY 1

*Bust/Chest*_____

*Waist*_____

*Hips*_____

MY DIET DIARY

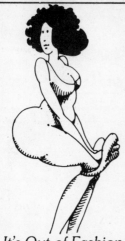

It's Out of Fashion To Be A Hippie!

THINK THIN SNACKS

Celebrate the end of a meal with a dessert coffee:

- add a stick of cinnamon
- rub an orange or lemon rind around the rim of your cup.
- steep two cloves in your cup
- lace the coffee with a teaspoon of brandy (11 calories) or dry sherry (7 calories)

A happy dieting story from the *1978 Guiness Book of World Records* is about Mrs. Celesta Geyer, the U.S. Circus Fat Lady. From 1950 to 1951, she lost an impressive 401 lbs., shrinking from 553 lbs. to 152 lbs. In December, 1967, 16 years after the diet, Mrs. Geyer was reported to weigh a tidy 110 lbs.

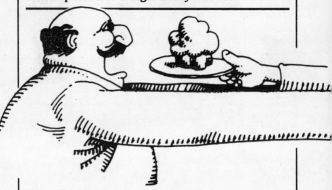

Over 99% of all people who are overweight are that way due to overeating and/or lack of exercise, and not because of hormonal imbalance, slow metabolic rate, heredity or "fat cells."

DAY 1

TODAY'S DATE [＿＿＿＿] **TODAY'S WEIGHT** [＿＿＿＿]

BREAKFAST ＿＿＿＿＿＿＿＿＿＿＿＿＿
＿＿＿＿＿＿＿＿＿＿＿＿＿＿＿＿＿＿＿
＿＿＿＿＿＿＿＿＿＿＿＿＿＿＿＿＿＿＿
＿＿＿ Calories

LUNCH ＿＿＿＿＿＿＿＿＿＿＿＿＿＿＿
＿＿＿＿＿＿＿＿＿＿＿＿＿＿＿＿＿＿＿
＿＿＿＿＿＿＿＿＿＿＿＿＿＿＿＿＿＿＿
＿＿＿＿＿＿＿＿＿＿＿＿＿＿＿＿＿＿＿
＿＿＿ Calories

DINNER ＿＿＿＿＿＿＿＿＿＿＿＿＿＿
＿＿＿＿＿＿＿＿＿＿＿＿＿＿＿＿＿＿＿
＿＿＿＿＿＿＿＿＿＿＿＿＿＿＿＿＿＿＿
＿＿＿＿＿＿＿＿＿＿＿＿＿＿＿＿＿＿＿
＿＿＿＿＿＿＿＿＿＿＿＿＿＿＿＿＿＿＿
＿＿＿ Calories

SNACKS ＿＿＿＿＿＿＿＿＿＿＿＿＿＿
＿＿＿＿＿＿＿＿＿＿＿＿＿＿＿＿＿＿＿
＿＿＿ Calories

EXERCISES ＿＿＿＿＿＿＿＿＿＿＿＿＿
＿＿＿＿＿＿＿＿＿＿＿＿＿＿＿＿＿＿＿
＿＿＿＿＿＿＿＿＿＿＿＿＿＿＿＿＿＿＿

FEATHERS IN MY CAP
(Triumphs Over Temptation)
＿＿＿＿＿＿＿＿＿
＿＿＿＿＿＿＿＿＿
＿＿＿＿＿＿＿＿＿
＿＿＿＿＿＿＿＿＿
＿＿＿＿＿＿＿＿＿

BLACK MARKS AGAINST ME
(Secret Splurges)
＿＿＿＿＿＿＿＿＿
＿＿＿＿＿＿＿＿＿
＿＿＿＿＿＿＿＿＿
＿＿＿＿＿＿＿＿＿
＿＿＿＿＿＿＿＿＿

MY DIET DIARY

A small green olive
has only 3 small calories.

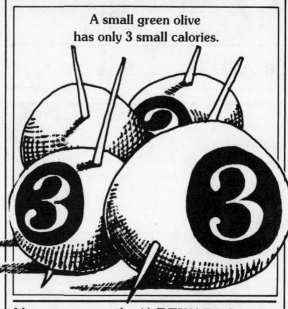

*You can eat until
you're stuffed, or
you can eat until
you're satisfied.
It's up to you.*

REWARDS

You won't have to
hide your tummy
when you wear a bikini.

Nuts are high in calories because they're high
in fat. Most nuts have about 800 calories per
cup. If you insist upon nuts, *you're nuts*!

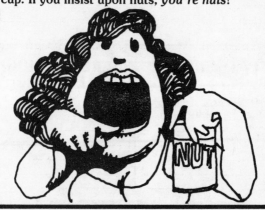

DAY 2

TODAY'S DATE		TODAY'S WEIGHT	

BREAKFAST _____
_____
_____
_____ Calories

LUNCH _____
_____
_____
_____
_____ Calories

DINNER _____
_____
_____
_____
_____
_____
_____ Calories

SNACKS _____
_____
_____
_____ Calories

EXERCISES _____
_____
_____
_____

FEATHERS IN MY CAP (Triumphs Over Temptation)	**BLACK MARKS AGAINST ME** (Secret Splurges)
_____	_____
_____	_____
_____	_____
_____	_____

MY DIET DIARY

In order to burn less gas, you should fill up your car's gas tank before it's half empty; likewise, in order to consume less calories, fill up your stomach with "think thin snacks" before it's empty and your hunger is out of control.

REWARDS

No more condescending remarks from family and friends about your "weight problem."

Think your waist is small enough? Queen Catherine di Medici (1519–89) decreed a standard waist measurement of 13 inches for all ladies of the French court.

NOBODY IS MAKING YOU EAT.

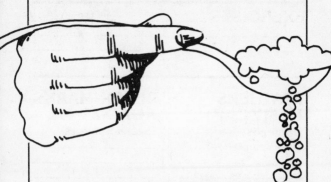

One tablespoon of grated parmesan cheese sprinkled on vegetables adds only 25 calories and lots of flavor.

DAY 3

TODAY'S DATE [   ]   **TODAY'S WEIGHT** [   ]

BREAKFAST _____
_____
_____
_____ Calories

LUNCH _____
_____
_____
_____
_____ Calories

DINNER _____
_____
_____
_____
_____
_____
_____ Calories

SNACKS _____
_____
_____
_____ Calories

EXERCISES _____
_____
_____

FEATHERS IN MY CAP (Triumphs Over Temptation)	**BLACK MARKS AGAINST ME** (Secret Splurges)
_____	_____
_____	_____
_____	_____
_____	_____

MY DIET DIARY

While most fruit pies divvy up into eight 300-calorie slices, strawberry pie has only 185 calories per slice. Recipe: Fill one prepared 9-inch pie crust with fresh strawberries. Heat ½ cup currant preserves until they become thin, and pour over berries. Chill and serve. Save even more calories by using dietetic preserves.

YOU BURN 2 CALORIES EVERY MINUTE YOU SPEND WRITING IN THIS DIARY.

Stuffing food in your mouth rarely makes you feel better about yourself, and those extra pounds will make you feel worse in the long run.

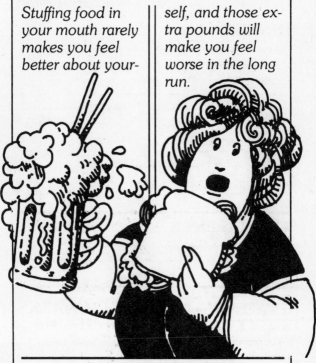

EAT LESS—SAVOR MORE.

Don't be unsociable—you can dine with others. Just take smaller portions and skip the sauces, salad dressing and sweet spreads.

DAY 4

TODAY'S DATE [ ]   **TODAY'S WEIGHT** [ ]

BREAKFAST _____
_____
_____
_____ Calories

LUNCH _____
_____
_____
_____
_____ Calories

DINNER _____
_____
_____
_____
_____
_____
_____ Calories

SNACKS _____
_____
_____
_____ Calories

EXERCISES _____
_____
_____
_____

FEATHERS IN MY CAP
(Triumphs Over Temptation)
_____
_____
_____
_____

BLACK MARKS AGAINST ME
(Secret Splurges)
_____
_____
_____
_____

17

MY DIET DIARY

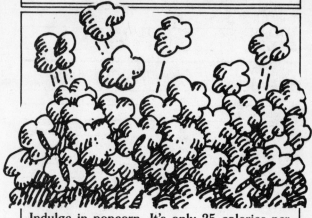

Indulge in popcorn. It's only 25 calories per cup if you skip the butter. Seasoned salt will bring out the flavor.

WHEN YOU GO TO THE SUPERMARKET, MAKE A SHOPPING LIST AND STICK TO IT.

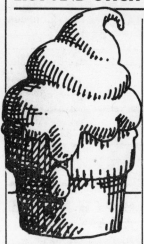

Ice cream is not Mt. Everest. You don't have to take it just because it's there.

Lunch at a deli? Sure! Order a tuna or salmon sandwich, made from a small, whole can of tuna, hold the mayo. Skip the potato salad and go for the kosher pickles.

THINK THIN SNACKS

Raw snap beans have plenty of crunch when you need to munch. They're only 30 calories a cup.

DAY 5

TODAY'S DATE		TODAY'S WEIGHT	

BREAKFAST _____
_____
_____
_____ Calories

LUNCH _____
_____
_____
_____
_____ Calories

DINNER _____
_____
_____
_____
_____
_____
_____ Calories

SNACKS _____
_____
_____
_____ Calories

EXERCISES _____
_____
_____
_____

FEATHERS IN MY CAP
(Triumphs Over Temptation)
_____
_____
_____
_____
_____

BLACK MARKS AGAINST ME
(Secret Splurges)
_____
_____
_____
_____
_____

MY DIET DIARY

If you can't re-member what a hunger pang feels like, you're eating according to the clock rather than according to your body.

If you skip the two tablespoons of may-onnaise in your cheese sandwich, your body is free of 220 calories which you *won't* have to run or sweat off, or fit your pants over.

Tight clothes may not look good on fat bodies, but a pinched belt, bulging buttons, and crease lines are great reminders to not pack in any more food.

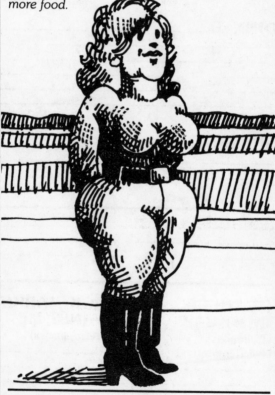

FEELING LOW ON ENERGY?
TAKE TWENTY DEEP BREATHS.

DAY 6

TODAY'S DATE [ ]   **TODAY'S WEIGHT** [ ]

BREAKFAST _____
_____
_____ Calories

LUNCH _____
_____
_____
_____ Calories

DINNER _____
_____
_____
_____
_____
_____ Calories

SNACKS _____
_____
_____ Calories

EXERCISES _____
_____
_____

FEATHERS IN MY CAP
(Triumphs Over Temptation)
_____
_____
_____
_____

BLACK MARKS AGAINST ME
(Secret Splurges)
_____
_____
_____
_____

21

MY DIET DIARY

THE TALLER YOU STAND, THE THINNER YOU LOOK.

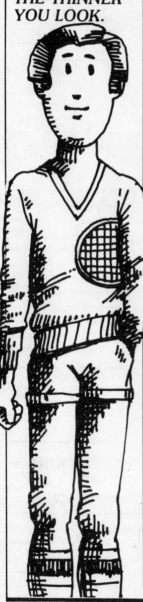

When your host is taking requests from the bar, ask for a mineral water or club soda with a twist of lime and save over a hundred calories. If you must drink, try a white wine spritzer or the ever popular Virgin Mary.

A THINNER, LIGHTER BODY REQUIRES LESS FOOD THAN A HEAVY ONE.

A steaming pot full of second helpings should go straight into the refrigerator for tomorrow's meal. Don't keep extra food in a serving bowl on the table right in front of your empty plate.

DAY 7

TODAY'S DATE [   ]   TODAY'S WEIGHT [   ]

BREAKFAST _____
_____
_____ ___ Calories

LUNCH _____
_____
_____
_____ ___ Calories

DINNER _____
_____
_____
_____
_____
_____ ___ Calories

SNACKS _____
_____
_____ ___ Calories

EXERCISES _____
_____
_____
_____

FEATHERS IN MY CAP
(Triumphs Over Temptation)
_____
_____
_____
_____

BLACK MARKS AGAINST ME
(Secret Splurges)
_____
_____
_____
_____

23

MY DIET DIARY

You can invite a dieter to a dinner party, but you can't make him eat.

THINK THIN SNACKS

If you can't stand to eat breakfast, then drink it. Blend 2 cups skim milk, a large banana, and protein powder for a 200-calorie, high energy milkshake.

Dining Italian style? Avoid the pasta and order a low-carbohydrate entrée like veal marsala. If you want something more, try a vegetable side dish.

LOOKING GOOD IS TANTAMOUNT TO FEELING GOOD.

No matter how much you eat, the feeling of hunger won't abate until twenty minutes after the start of a meal. Slow down over your appetizer until your appetite slows down with you.

The best time to stop a pig-out is at the idea stage.

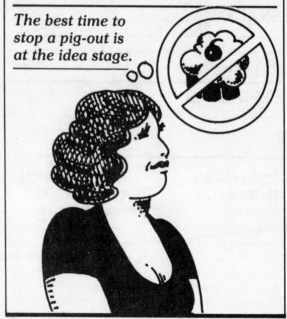

DAY 8

TODAY'S DATE		TODAY'S WEIGHT	

BREAKFAST _____

_____
_____
_____ ____ Calories

LUNCH _____

_____
_____
_____ ____ Calories

DINNER _____

_____
_____
_____
_____
_____ ____ Calories

SNACKS _____

_____
_____ ____ Calories

EXERCISES _____

_____
_____

FEATHERS IN MY CAP (Triumphs Over Temptation)	**BLACK MARKS AGAINST ME** (Secret Splurges)
_____	_____
_____	_____
_____	_____
_____	_____

25

MY DIET DIARY

Weigh yourself in the morning, before breakfast, when you're at your lightest. Let the results inspire you for the rest of the day.

WARNING: OVERWEIGHT MAY BE HAZARDOUS TO YOUR HEALTH.

Eating Chinese? Fill up on soup and tea, and ask your waiter not to bring you any rice.

Want to join a band? Playing drums burns calories twice as fast as playing the piano.

Next time you want to fill your stomach, fill the bathtub instead and relax in a delightful bubble bath.

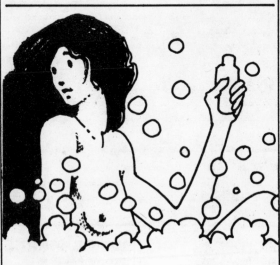

THINK BROIL, NOT FRY.

DAY 9

TODAY'S DATE [ ]   **TODAY'S WEIGHT** [ ]

BREAKFAST _____
_____
_____
_____ Calories

LUNCH _____
_____
_____
_____
_____ Calories

DINNER _____
_____
_____
_____
_____
_____
_____ Calories

SNACKS _____
_____
_____
_____ Calories

EXERCISES _____
_____
_____
_____

FEATHERS IN MY CAP
(Triumphs Over Temptation)
_____
_____
_____
_____

BLACK MARKS AGAINST ME
(Secret Splurges)
_____
_____
_____
_____

27

MY DIET DIARY

Some foods are high in calories and low in nutrients. These include butter, margarine, mayonnaise, candy, sugar, jam, syrups, alcohol, soda pop, refined breads, cakes, and cookies. AVOID THEM.

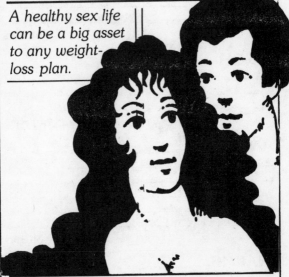

A healthy sex life can be a big asset to any weight-loss plan.

BUDGET WISELY. SAVE ON CALORIES AT REGULAR MEALS SO YOU CAN AFFORD TO SPEND THEM ON SPECIAL OCCASIONS.

A calorie is not the same calorie at breakfast and at dinner. It's a skinnier calorie in the morning.

Alcohol: What is it doing to you? The # of ounces *times* the proof *times* .8 *equals* the # of calories.

Lace your stews, sauces, meat, and sauteed veggies with wine or rum. They'll taste "richer" and 85 percent of the calories in the alcohol are burned off in three minutes of cooking. Season vegetables with herbs instead of flavoring them with rich sauces or fats.

DAY 10

TODAY'S DATE [ ]   **TODAY'S WEIGHT** [ ]

BREAKFAST _____
_____
_____
_____ ____ Calories

LUNCH _____
_____
_____
_____
_____ ____ Calories

DINNER _____
_____
_____
_____
_____
_____
_____ ____ Calories

SNACKS _____
_____
_____
_____ ____ Calories

EXERCISES _____
_____
_____
_____

FEATHERS IN MY CAP
(Triumphs Over Temptation)
_____
_____
_____
_____
_____

BLACK MARKS AGAINST ME
(Secret Splurges)
_____
_____
_____
_____
_____

MY DIET DIARY

Two cocktails before dinner? Did you know they fill one-quarter of your daily caloric needs!

Ask your friends for positive support rather than criticism.

SUGAR NOT ONLY MAKES YOU FAT, IT CAN MAKE YOU CRAZY. THE QUICK-ENERGY "BOOST" THAT SUGAR PROVIDES WEARS OFF QUICKLY, OFTEN LEAVING YOU EVEN MORE PHYSICALLY DEPLETED AND EMOTIONALLY DRAINED.

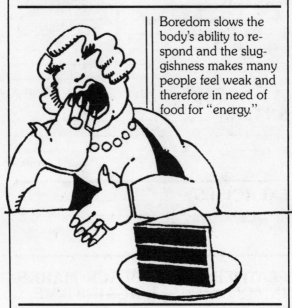

Boredom slows the body's ability to respond and the sluggishness makes many people feel weak and therefore in need of food for "energy."

WEIGHT MAINTENANCE FORMULA

Multiply your weight (in pounds) by **12** to get the number of calories you may consume each day in order to maintain your weight. Any more and you'll gain, any less and you'll lose.

DAY 11

TODAY'S DATE [   ]   TODAY'S WEIGHT [   ]

BREAKFAST _____
_____
_____
_____ Calories

LUNCH _____
_____
_____
_____
_____ Calories

DINNER _____
_____
_____
_____
_____
_____
_____ Calories

SNACKS _____
_____
_____
_____ Calories

EXERCISES _____
_____
_____

FEATHERS IN MY CAP
(Triumphs Over Temptation)
_____
_____
_____
_____
_____

BLACK MARKS AGAINST ME
(Secret Splurges)
_____
_____
_____
_____
_____

31

MY DIET DIARY

A frankfurter has 50 less calories than a hamburger, but frankfurter rolls have more calories than hamburger rolls!

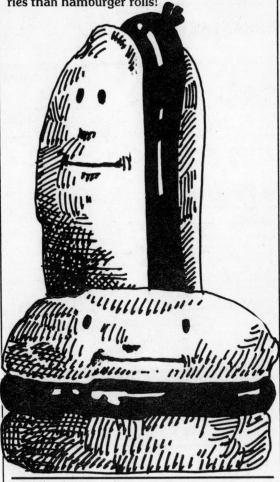

YOU CAN'T BE GORGEOUS IF YOU GORGE YOURSELF.

Next time you're contemplating a high-calorie snack, think of your lover and how you feel when he or she appreciates your body, and tell yourself, 'I don't need to eat this.''

DAY 12

TODAY'S DATE [____] **TODAY'S WEIGHT** [____]

BREAKFAST _____
_____
_____
_____ Calories

LUNCH _____
_____
_____
_____
_____ Calories

DINNER _____
_____
_____
_____
_____
_____
_____ Calories

SNACKS _____
_____
_____ Calories

EXERCISES _____
_____
_____
_____

FEATHERS IN MY CAP
(Triumphs Over Temptation)
_____
_____
_____
_____

BLACK MARKS AGAINST ME
(Secret Splurges)
_____
_____
_____
_____

33

MY DIET DIARY

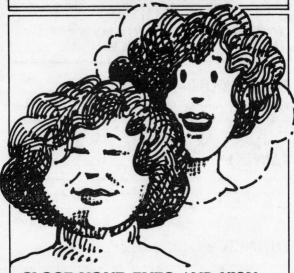

CLOSE YOUR EYES AND VISU-
ALIZE YOURSELF BECOMING
SLIMMER.

You'll have a lot
more room in
your pocketbook
if you don't carry
a candy bar
around all the
time.

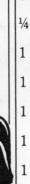

THINK THIN SNACKS

1 2" plum: 30 cal.
1 large stalk celery: 5 cal.
¼ head lettuce: 13 cal.
1 c. steamed spin-ach: 26 cal.
1 c. summer squash: 35 cal.
1 c. watercress: 9 cal.
1 c. strawberries: 54 cal.
1 c. bean sprouts: 17 cal.
1 c. coffee, black: 3 cal.
1 c. unsweetened tea: 4 cal.

DAY 13

TODAY'S DATE [　　]　　**TODAY'S WEIGHT** [　　]

BREAKFAST _____
_____
_____
_____ ____ Calories

LUNCH _____
_____
_____
_____
_____ ____ Calories

DINNER _____
_____
_____
_____
_____
_____
_____ ____ Calories

SNACKS _____
_____
_____
_____ ____ Calories

EXERCISES _____
_____
_____
_____

FEATHERS IN MY CAP
(Triumphs Over Temptation)
_____
_____
_____
_____
_____

BLACK MARKS AGAINST ME
(Secret Splurges)
_____
_____
_____
_____
_____

MY DIET DIARY

It's easy to forget about food when you're involved in helping other people. Join a volunteer program.

THINK THIN SNACKS

Cut a raw zucchini into slivers and sprinkle with seasoned salt. A half-cup is only 11 calories.

When your waitress asks what you'll have to drink, it's okay to order a glass of ice water with a twist of lemon.

Adding milk to egg batter toughens the eggs and makes them more caloric. Scramble your eggs with a little cold water.

Steambaths are not only sensual, they (temporarily) remove excess pounds.

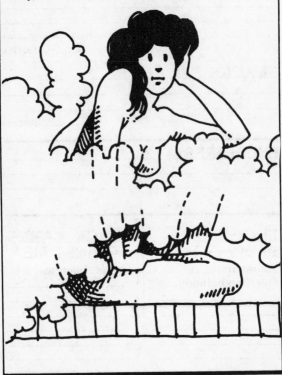

DAY 14

TODAY'S DATE [   ]   **TODAY'S WEIGHT** [   ]

BREAKFAST _____
_____
_____
_____ ____ Calories

LUNCH _____
_____
_____
_____
_____ ____ Calories

DINNER _____
_____
_____
_____
_____
_____ ____ Calories

SNACKS _____
_____
_____
_____ ____ Calories

EXERCISES _____
_____
_____
_____

FEATHERS IN MY CAP
(Triumphs Over Temptation)
_____
_____
_____
_____

BLACK MARKS AGAINST ME
(Secret Splurges)
_____
_____
_____
_____

MY DIET DIARY

At McDonald's, plain scrambled eggs have half the calories of an Egg McMuffin.

One good-sized slice of Boston Cream Pie has half your daily calories in it.

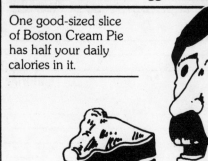

REWARDS

You'll not only look younger, you'll feel younger.

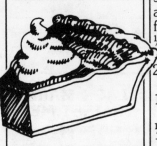

Any Pie Is Fattening—Any Way You Slice It.

THINK THIN SNACKS

Some foods, thought of as fattening, are not so in unadulterated and/or moderate form:

½ an average lobster: 92 calories
2 slices bacon: 95 cal.
1 tsp. French dressing: 20 cal.
½ cup wine: 100 cal.
1 caramel candy: 21 cal.
1 tsp. sugar: 17 cal.
2″ × 2″ × ½″ slice of fruit cake: 105 cal.

DAY 15

TODAY'S DATE [ ]　**TODAY'S WEIGHT** [ ]

BREAKFAST _____
_____
_____
_____ Calories

LUNCH _____
_____
_____
_____
_____ Calories

DINNER _____
_____
_____
_____
_____
_____ Calories

SNACKS _____
_____
_____
_____ Calories

EXERCISES _____
_____
_____
_____

FEATHERS IN MY CAP
(Triumphs Over Temptation)
_____
_____
_____
_____

BLACK MARKS AGAINST ME
(Secret Splurges)
_____
_____
_____
_____

39

MY DIET DIARY

THERE'S NOTHING HEROIC ABOUT EATING A HERO.

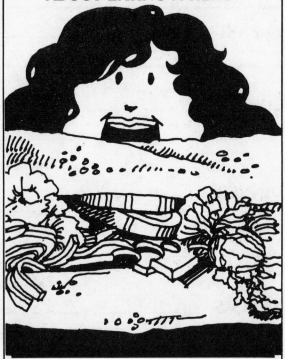

For low-calorie dips and salad dressings, substitute low-fat yogurt for sour cream and save 360 calories per cup.

If you've had a lapse in your diet, the first thing you must do is forgive yourself.

The amount of fat on a 3-ounce broiled steak can double its caloric content.

Stamp out psychological starvation: Eat bulky (low-calorie) green vegetables.

Graciously accept dinner invitations and assure your hostess you'll eat anything, but in small portions. That way she won't take it personally if you don't eat heartily.

DAY 16

TODAY'S DATE [ ] **TODAY'S WEIGHT** [ ]

BREAKFAST _____

_____

_____
_____ Calories

LUNCH _____

_____

_____

_____
_____ Calories

DINNER _____

_____

_____

_____

_____

_____
_____ Calories

SNACKS _____

_____

_____
_____ Calories

EXERCISES _____

_____

_____

_____

FEATHERS IN MY CAP
(Triumphs Over Temptation)

BLACK MARKS AGAINST ME
(Secret Splurges)

41

MY DIET DIARY

As soon as you sit down in a restaurant order a relish tray. The radishes and carrot sticks will busy your hands and keep them out of the bread basket.

NO DIET WILL WORK FOR YOU IF YOU DON'T WORK ON THE DIET.

THINK THIN SNACKS

Desperate for sweets? Marshmallows are a mixture of 23 calories and a lot of air.

Small lady fingers are a ladylike 18 calories.

Don't be fooled: Frozen yogurt has 135–150 calories per half-cup; supermarket-style ice cream has less.

Three dates have only 50 calories.

Cocoa made with three ounces of milk and three ounces of water—and no sugar—has only 100 calories.

Stick a half-grapefruit under the broiler for five minutes, sprinkle with cinamon, and you'll get a sticky, sweet, 50-calorie dessert.

REWARDS

You'll look forward to bathing suit weather.

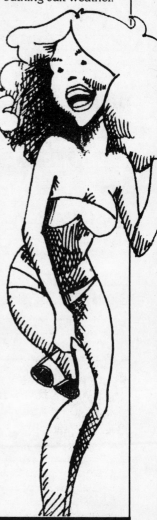

DAY 17

TODAY'S DATE		TODAY'S WEIGHT	

BREAKFAST _____

_____

_____ ____ Calories

LUNCH _____ ___

_____ _____ ___

_____ ___

_____ ____ Calories

DINNER _____

_____

_____

_____

_____

_____ ____ Calories

SNACKS _____

_____

_____ ____ Calories

EXERCISES _____

_____

_____

FEATHERS IN MY CAP (Triumphs Over Temptation)	BLACK MARKS AGAINST ME (Secret Splurges)
_____	_____
_____	_____
_____	_____
_____	_____

43

MY DIET DIARY

Over the course of a lifetime, the average eater takes about 4 million bites of food. You could do without a few hundred of them.

DIETING IS THE ONE GAME IN WHICH LOSERS WIN AND GAINERS LOSE.

DAY 18

TODAY'S DATE [ ] **TODAY'S WEIGHT** [ ]

BREAKFAST _____
_____
_____
_____ ____ Calories

LUNCH _____
_____
_____
_____
_____ ____ Calories

DINNER _____
_____
_____
_____
_____
_____ ____ Calories

SNACKS _____
_____
_____
_____ ____ Calories

EXERCISES _____
_____
_____
_____

FEATHERS IN MY CAP
(Triumphs Over Temptation)
_____
_____
_____
_____

BLACK MARKS AGAINST ME
(Secret Splurges)
_____
_____
_____
_____

MY DIET DIARY

THINK THIN SNACKS

Place one slice of low-fat cheese on a slice of high fiber toast. When the cheese is melted, place a second slice of toast on top. Calories: 325 (versus 525 for a regular grilled-cheese sandwich)

Wrong: "I won't eat rich dessert."
Right: "I <u>don't</u> eat rich desserts."

Instead of putting food in your mouth just now, try kissing some-one!

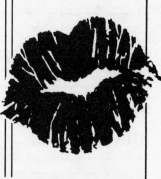

The sex act burns about 150 calories.

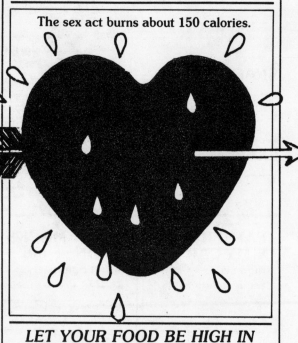

LET YOUR FOOD BE HIGH IN QUALITY, NOT QUANTITY.

DAY 19

TODAY'S DATE		TODAY'S WEIGHT	

BREAKFAST _____
_____
_____
_____ ____ Calories

LUNCH _____
_____
_____
_____
_____ ____ Calories

DINNER _____
_____
_____
_____
_____
_____
_____ ____ Calories

SNACKS _____
_____
_____
_____ ____ Calories

EXERCISES _____
_____
_____
_____

FEATHERS IN MY CAP (Triumphs Over Temptation)	**BLACK MARKS AGAINST ME** (Secret Splurges)
_____	_____
_____	_____
_____	_____
_____	_____

47

MY DIET DIARY

For business lunches where you have to "keep up" with your clients, pre-arrange with the waiter to bring you straight ginger-ale every time you order another round of drinks for the table.

CHEATING ON YOUR DIET IS NOT A "VICTIMLESS" CRIME.

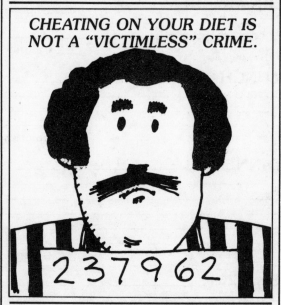

It's okay to tell the waiter to bring the check right after the main course and to not ask if you'd like any dessert.

If you're near something that smells irresistible, MOVE AWAY FROM IT.

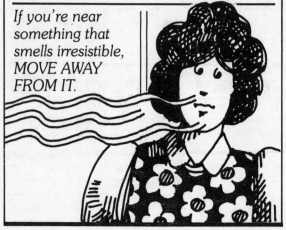

DAY 20

TODAY'S DATE [   ] TODAY'S WEIGHT [   ]

BREAKFAST _____
_____
_____
_____ ____ Calories

LUNCH _____
_____
_____
_____ ____ Calories

DINNER _____
_____
_____
_____
_____
_____ ____ Calories

SNACKS _____
_____
_____ ____ Calories

EXERCISES _____
_____
_____

FEATHERS IN MY CAP
(Triumphs Over Temptation)
_____
_____
_____
_____

BLACK MARKS AGAINST ME
(Secret Splurges)
_____
_____
_____
_____

49

MY DIET DIARY

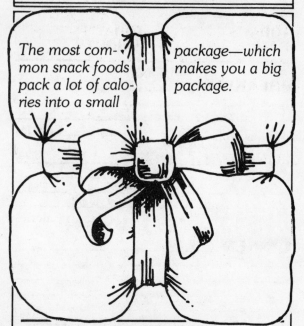

The most common snack foods pack a lot of calories into a small package—which makes you a big package.

POWDERED CREAMERS ARE JUST AS FATTENING AS DAIRY CREAM.

The older you get, the less you need to eat. With each birthday after 21, decrease ten calories from your daily intake.

ONLY IF NECESSARY

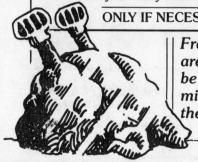

Frozen leftovers are less likely to be eaten during midnight raids to the refrigerator.

DAY 21

TODAY'S DATE [   ] **TODAY'S WEIGHT** [   ]

BREAKFAST _____
_____
_____
_____ ____ Calories

LUNCH _____
_____
_____
_____
_____ ____ Calories

DINNER _____
_____
_____
_____
_____
_____ ____ Calories

SNACKS _____
_____
_____
_____ ____ Calories

EXERCISES _____
_____
_____
_____

FEATHERS IN MY CAP
(Triumphs Over Temptation)

_____
_____
_____
_____

BLACK MARKS AGAINST ME
(Secret Splurges)

_____
_____
_____
_____

51

MY DIET DIARY

Numerous tests have found that people who eat their main meal early in the day lose more weight than those who consume an equal number of calories later in the day.

Depress your appetite with acupressure: Place your finger over your upper lip, just under your nose, and press upwards gently but firmly.

Variety is the spice of life. Flavor your diet with it.

NEED TO PUT SOMETHING SWEET IN YOUR MOUTH? TRY A TOOTHBRUSH.

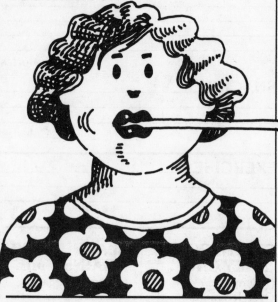

In general, a serving of fish or seafood has approximately half the calories of a serving of beef, lamb or pork. And a serving of vegetables has approximately one quarter of the calories of a serving of fish.

DAY 22

TODAY'S DATE [　　　]   TODAY'S WEIGHT [　　　]

BREAKFAST _____
_____
_____
_____ ___ Calories

LUNCH _____
_____
_____
_____
_____ ___ Calories

DINNER _____
_____
_____
_____
_____
_____
_____ ___ Calories

SNACKS _____
_____
_____
_____ ___ Calories

EXERCISES _____
_____
_____
_____

FEATHERS IN MY CAP
(Triumphs Over Temptation)
_____
_____
_____
_____

BLACK MARKS AGAINST ME
(Secret Splurges)
_____
_____
_____
_____

53

MY DIET DIARY

THINK THIN SNACKS

Cucumbers, cauliflower, celery, kohlrabi, peppers, lettuce, endive, watercress, carrots, broccoli, zucchini, tomatoes, and spinach contain very few calories and a great many minerals and vitamins. They can fill you up when you're feeling empty.

The difference between thin people and fat people is that thin people can live with the sensation of an empty stomach and fat people can't.

In filling a hungry stomach, WATER is rarely given enough respect.

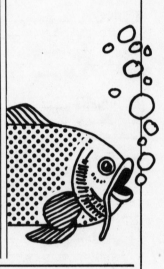

Non-dairy frozen creamer has just as many calories as half-and-half (30 per tablespoon).

Busy people rarely think about eating.

DAY 23

TODAY'S DATE [   ]   TODAY'S WEIGHT [   ]

BREAKFAST _____
_____
_____
_____ ___ Calories

LUNCH _____
_____
_____
_____
_____ ___ Calories

DINNER _____
_____
_____
_____
_____
_____
_____ ___ Calories

SNACKS _____
_____
_____
_____ ___ Calories

EXERCISES _____
_____
_____
_____

FEATHERS IN MY CAP (Triumphs Over Temptation)	**BLACK MARKS AGAINST ME** (Secret Splurges)
_____	_____
_____	_____
_____	_____
_____	_____

55

MY DIET DIARY

Studies have shown that fat people take bigger bites and chew less than thin people.

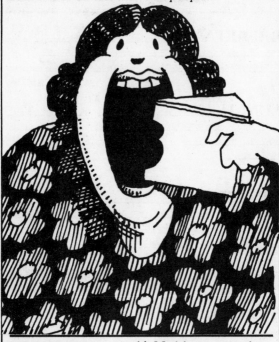

REWARDS

A new feeling of self-confidence.

THINK THIN SNACKS

Cold Curry Cucumber Soup:
Mix ½ tsp. ground cumin and ½ tsp. salt into a pint of low-fat yogurt and beat until frothy. Add one cucumber that's been peeled and diced. Calories: 125 per 1 cup serving.

Holding onto the perfect weight is a balancing act.

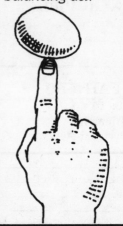

DAY 24

TODAY'S DATE		TODAY'S WEIGHT	

BREAKFAST _____
_____
_____
_____ Calories

LUNCH _____
_____
_____
_____
_____ Calories

DINNER _____
_____
_____
_____
_____
_____ Calories

SNACKS _____
_____
_____
_____ Calories

EXERCISES _____
_____
_____
_____

FEATHERS IN MY CAP (Triumphs Over Temptation)	**BLACK MARKS AGAINST ME** (Secret Splurges)
_____	_____
_____	_____
_____	_____
_____	_____

MY DIET DIARY

Exercise not only burns up calories, it has a calming effect and lowers the likelihood that you'll eat out of nervous frustration.

THINK THIN SNACKS

Whip up some dietetic jello in the morning to have later in the day. You can do it while your tea is brewing.

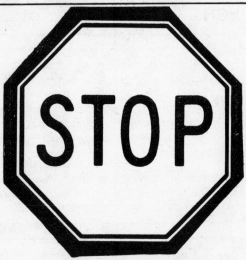

STOP OVEREATING

SMALL BITES TASTE AS GOOD AS BIG ONES.

REWARDS

Enjoying that feeling of power when you realize that you aren't a slave to food any-more.

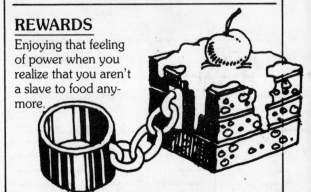

DAY 25

TODAY'S DATE [   ]   TODAY'S WEIGHT [   ]

BREAKFAST _____
_____
_____
_____ Calories

LUNCH _____
_____
_____
_____
_____ Calories

DINNER _____
_____
_____
_____
_____
_____
_____ Calories

SNACKS _____
_____
_____
_____ Calories

EXERCISES _____
_____
_____
_____

FEATHERS IN MY CAP
(Triumphs Over Temptation)
_____
_____
_____
_____

BLACK MARKS AGAINST ME
(Secret Splurges)
_____
_____
_____
_____

MY DIET DIARY

WINNING THE LOSING BATTLE CALLS FOR LOTS OF PERSEVER- ANCE, BUT IT CAN BE DONE.

The more fat you keep around you, the farther it keeps people away from you.

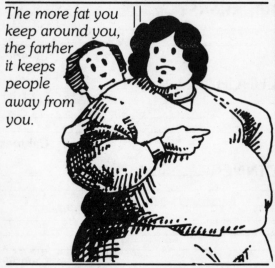

You have to walk for over *two hours* to burn off the calories eaten (in one minute) in one piece of chocolate cake. You can swim one full hour, and still not burn off the calories in **16 almonds.**

Skipping meals often leads to unplanned snacks, which leads to more calories.

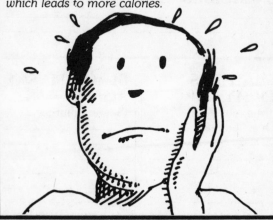

DAY 26

TODAY'S DATE [   ]   TODAY'S WEIGHT [   ]

BREAKFAST _____
_____
_____
_____ Calories

LUNCH _____
_____
_____
_____
_____ Calories

DINNER _____
_____
_____
_____
_____
_____
_____ Calories

SNACKS _____
_____
_____
_____ Calories

EXERCISES _____
_____
_____

FEATHERS IN MY CAP
(Triumphs Over Temptation)
_____
_____
_____
_____
_____

BLACK MARKS AGAINST ME
(Secret Splurges)
_____
_____
_____
_____
_____

61

MY DIET DIARY

Every morning look carefully at your naked body in the mirror and reaffirm your commitment to making it beautiful.

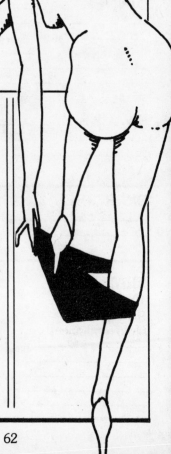

Sugar for "quick energy" stimulates the appetite so that you crave more food.

Lettuce leaves and parsley can make a plate look abundant without an abundance of calories.

The next time you are drawn uncontrollably into your kitchen, clean up your stove instead of cleaning out your refrigerator.

DAY 27

TODAY'S DATE [   ]   **TODAY'S WEIGHT** [   ]

BREAKFAST _____
_____
_____
_____ Calories

LUNCH _____
_____
_____
_____
_____ Calories

DINNER _____
_____
_____
_____
_____
_____ Calories

SNACKS _____
_____
_____
_____ Calories

EXERCISES _____
_____
_____

FEATHERS IN MY CAP
(Triumphs Over Temptation)
_____
_____
_____
_____
_____

BLACK MARKS AGAINST ME
(Secret Splurges)
_____
_____
_____
_____
_____

MY DIET DIARY

Cut your food into tiny morsels. It will help you eat more slowly—even the process of cutting takes time.

The weight that is best for you in your mid-twenties is best for you in your later years.

Someone passes you the hors d'oeuvres plate? Sure! Grab a radish from it.

THINK THIN SNACKS

Strong tasting foods go a long way to satisfying a flavor craving. Snack on as much of these foods as you like: sauerkraut, scallions, watercress, lemon, clam juice, dill pickles, endive, onion, parsley, and lime.

PEACE OF MIND CANNOT BE FOUND INSIDE A COOKIE JAR.

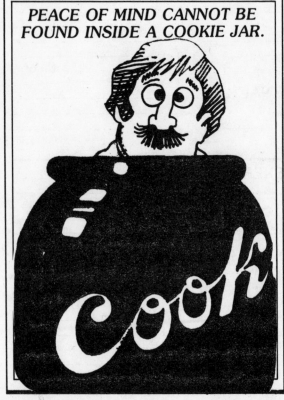

DAY 28

TODAY'S DATE [ ] **TODAY'S WEIGHT** [ ]

BREAKFAST _____
_____
_____
_____ Calories

LUNCH _____
_____
_____
_____ Calories

DINNER _____
_____
_____
_____
_____
_____ Calories

SNACKS _____
_____
_____
_____ Calories

EXERCISES _____
_____
_____

FEATHERS IN MY CAP
(Triumphs Over Temptation)
_____
_____
_____
_____
_____

BLACK MARKS AGAINST ME
(Secret Splurges)
_____
_____
_____
_____
_____

65

MY DIET DIARY

Whatever you're angry about, don't take it out on your body. Don't eat, punch a pillow instead.

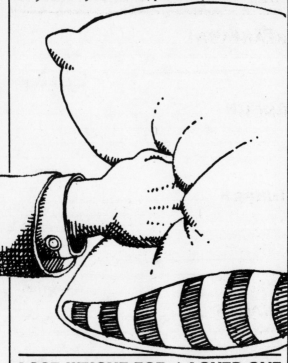

LOSE WEIGHT FOR A LOVED ONE —YOURSELF!

In order to lose one pound a week, you must cut your calorie intake by 500 a day.

Anything in your stomach will make you feel less hungry when you sit down to eat. Have a before-dinner glass of water or cup of bouillon.

THINK THIN SNACKS

Dessert? A cup of whole fresh strawberries has less than a hundred calories. Relish them.

DAY 29

TODAY'S DATE [   ]   TODAY'S WEIGHT [   ]

BREAKFAST _____
_____
_____
_____ ___ Calories

LUNCH _____
_____
_____
_____
_____ ___ Calories

DINNER _____
_____
_____
_____
_____
_____
_____ ___ Calories

SNACKS _____
_____
_____
_____ ___ Calories

EXERCISES _____
_____
_____
_____

FEATHERS IN MY CAP (Triumphs Over Temptation)	BLACK MARKS AGAINST ME (Secret Splurges)
_____	_____
_____	_____
_____	_____
_____	_____
_____	_____

MY DIET DIARY

THINK THIN SNACKS

Jazz up tomato juice with Worcestershire sauce, red pepper sauce, lemon juice and a grating of fresh pepper or a sprinkling of fresh chives. Calories: 50 per 8-ounce glass.

When you're active, you not only burn more calories, you can get more things accomplished.

Keep an abundant supply of "think-thin snacks" ready to serve in the refrigerator, so you'll reach for them instead of anything more destructive.

A mid-morning snack of half a grapefruit will curb your hunger at lunch.

Take up a hobby. It's hard to play the saxophone and eat at the same time.

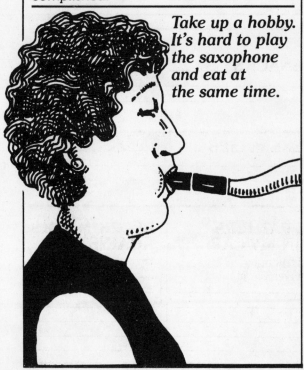

DAY 30

TODAY'S DATE [____] TODAY'S WEIGHT [____]

BREAKFAST _____
_____
_____
_____ Calories

LUNCH _____
_____
_____
_____
_____ Calories

DINNER _____
_____
_____
_____
_____
_____
_____ Calories

SNACKS _____
_____
_____ Calories

EXERCISES _____
_____
_____
_____

FEATHERS IN MY CAP
(Triumphs Over Temptation)
_____
_____
_____
_____

BLACK MARKS AGAINST ME
(Secret Splurges)
_____
_____
_____
_____

FULL LENGTH PHOTO
DAY 30

*Bust/Chest*_____

*Waist*_____

*Hips*_____

MY DIET DIARY

The fewer calories you consume, the harder it is to get the minerals and vitamins you need, so make each calorie count.

IF YOU EAT ON THE RUN, YOU RUN THE RISK OF OVEREATING.

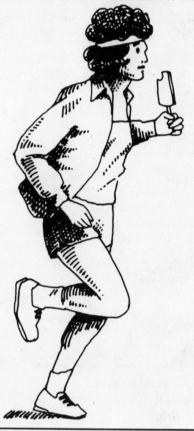

THINK THIN SNACKS

Fresh, raw spinach and mushrooms, without any dressing, make marvelous finger food.

You will be alive tomorrow. There's no need to eat every meal as though it were your last.

DAY 31

TODAY'S DATE ☐ **TODAY'S WEIGHT** ☐

BREAKFAST _____
_____
_____
_____ Calories

LUNCH _____
_____
_____
_____
_____ Calories

DINNER _____
_____
_____
_____
_____
_____
_____ Calories

SNACKS _____
_____
_____
_____ Calories

EXERCISES _____
_____
_____
_____

FEATHERS IN MY CAP (Triumphs Over Temptation)	**BLACK MARKS AGAINST ME** (Secret Splurges)

MY DIET DIARY

Drink all night, and only consume 100 calories: When your cocktail glass is half empty, fill 'er up with seltzer, and when that's half empty, fill 'er up again.

FEELING BLUE? REACH FOR THE PHONE INSTEAD OF THE FRIDGE.

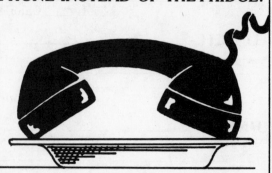

One can have conversations that are just as long, intimate, and wonderful while walking with a friend as one can have while eating with a friend.

Breakfast muffins such as corn, bran, and blueberry average 120 calories each—before the butter.

Instead of eating: Close your eyes, say "deep relaxation," and take three deep breaths.

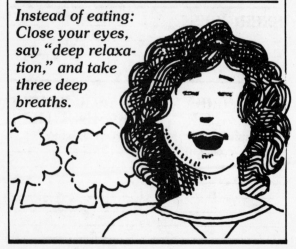

DAY 32

| TODAY'S DATE | | TODAY'S WEIGHT | |

BREAKFAST _____
_____
_____
_____ Calories

LUNCH _____
_____
_____
_____
_____ Calories

DINNER _____
_____
_____
_____
_____
_____
_____ Calories

SNACKS _____
_____
_____
_____ Calories

EXERCISES _____
_____
_____
_____

FEATHERS IN MY CAP (Triumphs Over Temptation)	**BLACK MARKS AGAINST ME** (Secret Splurges)
_____	_____
_____	_____
_____	_____
_____	_____

MY DIET DIARY

Beware of mechanical munching: It can happen to you anywhere —at the movies, while you're on the phone, in front of TV, or in your bed while you're reading.

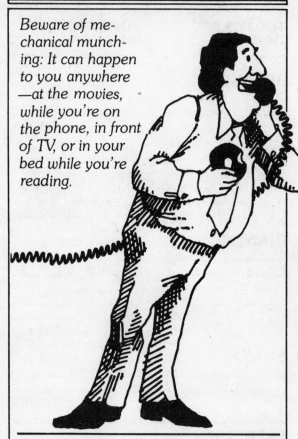

Instead of butter or margarine, dress up steamed vegetables with plain, low-fat yogurt and herbs.

A slice of toast has half the calories of a plain muffin.

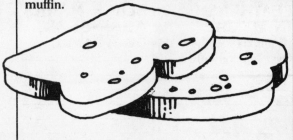

DAY 33

TODAY'S DATE [ ] **TODAY'S WEIGHT** [ ]

BREAKFAST _____
_____
_____
_____ Calories

LUNCH _____
_____
_____
_____
_____ Calories

DINNER _____
_____
_____
_____
_____
_____
_____ Calories

SNACKS _____
_____
_____
_____ Calories

EXERCISES _____
_____
_____
_____

FEATHERS IN MY CAP
(Triumphs Over Temptation)
_____
_____
_____
_____

BLACK MARKS AGAINST ME
(Secret Splurges)
_____
_____
_____
_____
_____

77

MY DIET DIARY

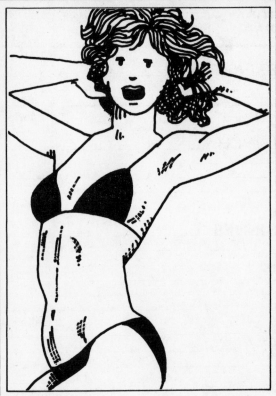

Instead of rewarding yourself with a cheeseburger, treat yourself with tickets to a concert, a new set of sexy underwear, or a long-distance call to a friend.

Need to take a food break from the work you're doing? Instead, put some great music on the stereo, stretch out on the floor or bed, and drink up the sounds.

THINK THIN SNACKS

Chocolate Rum Balls: Mix 1 package chocolate Alba 77 with ¼-cup water and 1½ tsp. rum flavor. Roll into cherry-size balls and freeze. Calories: Approx. 7 per candy.

DAY 34

TODAY'S
DATE [   ]

TODAY'S
WEIGHT [   ]

BREAKFAST _____

_____

_____

_____ Calories

LUNCH _____

_____

_____

_____

_____ Calories

DINNER _____

_____

_____

_____

_____

_____

_____ Calories

SNACKS _____

_____

_____

_____ Calories

EXERCISES _____

_____

_____

_____

FEATHERS IN MY CAP
(Triumphs Over Temptation)

_____

_____

_____

_____

_____

BLACK MARKS AGAINST ME
(Secret Splurges)

_____

_____

_____

_____

_____

MY DIET DIARY

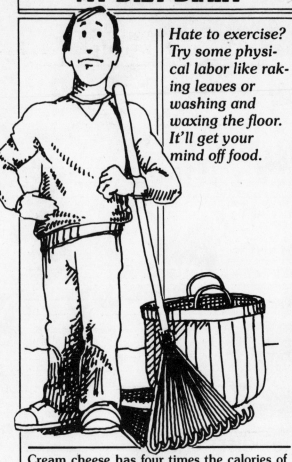

Hate to exercise? Try some physical labor like raking leaves or washing and waxing the floor. It'll get your mind off food.

Cream cheese has four times the calories of cottage cheese. Substitute often, and do only ¼ of the harm!

Fresh lemon sparks up vegetables, fish, and seafood. Who needs to dip lobster in butter?

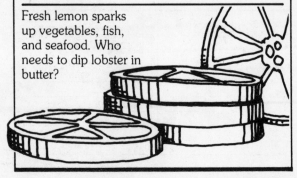

DAY 35

TODAY'S DATE [   ]   TODAY'S WEIGHT [   ]

BREAKFAST _____
_____
_____
_____ ___ Calories

LUNCH _____
_____
_____
_____
_____ ___ Calories

DINNER _____
_____
_____
_____
_____
_____ ___ Calories

SNACKS _____
_____
_____
_____ ___ Calories

EXERCISES _____
_____
_____
_____

FEATHERS IN MY CAP (Triumphs Over Temptation)	BLACK MARKS AGAINST ME (Secret Splurges)
_____	_____
_____	_____
_____	_____
_____	_____

MY DIET DIARY

A century ago it was a sign of affluence to have a wide girth. Today it's a sign of weakness.

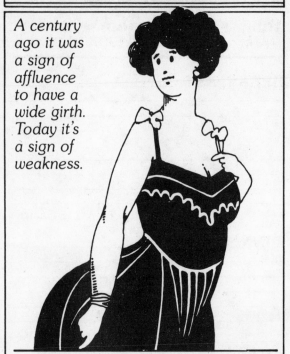

A "FAT CHANCE" IS NO CHANCE

A good way to not offend your host at a dinner party is to help yourself to small portions of food, but spread them over the entire surface of your plate. No one will notice your thin intentions.

REWARDS
Your heart will thank you.

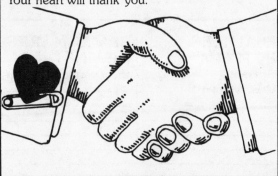

DAY 36

TODAY'S DATE [ ] **TODAY'S WEIGHT** [ ]

BREAKFAST _____
_____
_____
_____ ___ Calories

LUNCH _____
_____
_____
_____
_____ ___ Calories

DINNER _____
_____
_____
_____
_____
_____
_____ ___ Calories

SNACKS _____
_____
_____
_____ ___ Calories

EXERCISES _____
_____
_____
_____

FEATHERS IN MY CAP
(Triumphs Over Temptation)
_____
_____
_____
_____
_____

BLACK MARKS AGAINST ME
(Secret Splurges)
_____
_____
_____
_____
_____

MY DIET DIARY

Eating with chopsticks is good for your diet—especially when you aren't good with chopsticks.

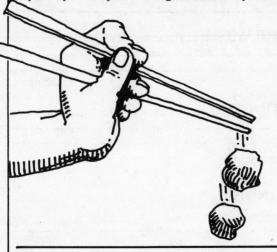

If you eat your main meal of the day at 5 or 6 P.M., you'll gain less weight than if you eat the exact same meal at 8 or 9 P.M.

Barbeque or broil your meats. Much of the fat drips down into the coals or broiler pan—and not into your stomach.

Disco dancing burns up as many calories as swimming (700 an hour). Why not do both.

THINK THIN SNACKS

For variety make ice tea from herbal teas. There are about thirty different flavors on the market, they have no calories, and they taste unique.

Give your taste buds a treat (and refresh your breath)—suck on a clove or a cardamom seed.

Shop with care. Steak that has lines of fat running through it will put lines of fat on you.

DAY 37

TODAY'S DATE [   ]   **TODAY'S WEIGHT** [   ]

BREAKFAST _____
_____
_____
_____ ___ Calories

LUNCH _____
_____
_____
_____
_____ ___ Calories

DINNER _____
_____
_____
_____
_____
_____
_____ ___ Calories

SNACKS _____
_____
_____
_____ ___ Calories

EXERCISES _____
_____
_____
_____

FEATHERS IN MY CAP
(Triumphs Over Temptation)
_____
_____
_____
_____
_____

BLACK MARKS AGAINST ME
(Secret Splurges)
_____
_____
_____
_____
_____

MY DIET DIARY

THINK THIN SNACKS

Substitute low-fat yogurt as a sandwich spread. Two tablespoons of low-fat yogurt = 16 calories. (Two tablespoons of mayonnaise = 202 calories.)

Before you head for the refrigerator, do three minutes of exercise and take a good assessment of the shape you're in.

FIBER?

Think it only comes in bran? You can get *twice* the fiber of a bran muffin in 3½ oz. of raw blueberries, cooked lentils, beans or mushrooms. One artichoke has *four* times more fiber than the muffin.

A QUART OF WATER A DAY KEEPS THE HUNGRIES AWAY.

REWARDS

Looking and feeling sexier.

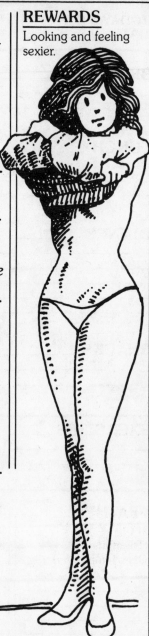

DAY 38

TODAY'S DATE [   ] TODAY'S WEIGHT [   ]

BREAKFAST _____
_____
_____
_____ ____ Calories

LUNCH _____
_____
_____
_____
_____ ____ Calories

DINNER _____
_____
_____
_____
_____
_____
_____ ____ Calories

SNACKS _____
_____
_____
_____ ____ Calories

EXERCISES _____
_____
_____
_____

FEATHERS IN MY CAP
(Triumphs Over Temptation)
_____
_____
_____
_____
_____

BLACK MARKS AGAINST ME
(Secret Splurges)
_____
_____
_____
_____
_____

87

MY DIET DIARY

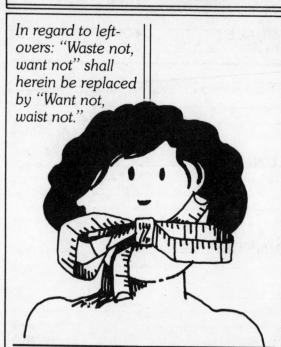

In regard to leftovers: "Waste not, want not" shall herein be replaced by "Want not, waist not."

TAKE THE TIME TO TASTE WHAT YOU'RE EATING.

Diet device for those who can't give up snacks: eat only between meals.

A hard candy has less than half the calories of a chocolate kiss, and the sweet pleasure lasts ten times as long.

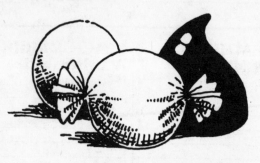

DAY 39

TODAY'S DATE [   ]   **TODAY'S WEIGHT** [   ]

BREAKFAST _____
_____
_____
_____ Calories

LUNCH _____
_____
_____
_____ Calories

DINNER _____
_____
_____
_____
_____
_____ Calories

SNACKS _____
_____
_____ Calories

EXERCISES _____
_____
_____

FEATHERS IN MY CAP
(Triumphs Over Temptation)
_____
_____
_____
_____

BLACK MARKS AGAINST ME
(Secret Splurges)
_____
_____
_____
_____

MY DIET DIARY

In today's competitive world, a slim, trim body is often taken to reflect a winning attitude.

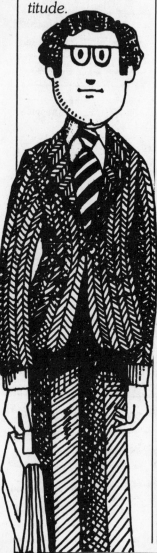

REWARDS

You won't have to worry about having the right clothes to wear.

When dining out choose a Chinese or Japanese restaurant where you won't be tempted by warm bread baskets or sumptuous dessert trays.

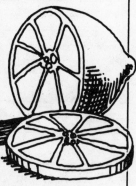

Lemon and lime can really jazz up a glass of water or club soda.

THINK THIN SNACKS

Run raw carrots through the thinnest crinkle-cut blade of a food processor and munch on carrot chips instead of potato chips.

DAY 40

TODAY'S DATE [　　　] **TODAY'S WEIGHT** [　　　]

BREAKFAST _____
_____
_____
_____ ____ Calories

LUNCH _____
_____
_____
_____
_____ ____ Calories

DINNER _____
_____
_____
_____
_____
_____
_____ ____ Calories

SNACKS _____
_____
_____
_____ ____ Calories

EXERCISES _____
_____
_____
_____

FEATHERS IN MY CAP (Triumphs Over Temptation)	**BLACK MARKS AGAINST ME** (Secret Splurges)
_____	_____
_____	_____
_____	_____
_____	_____
_____	_____

MY DIET DIARY

Skipping a meal can cause headache, weakness and tension, which often result in a binge at the next meal.

The natural taste of food is yours to enjoy when you stop consuming artificial sweeteners.

After-dinner cordials are not all equal. Eighty-proof brandy has 67 calories per ounce, curacao has 72, apricot brandy has 81. Creme de menthe has 105.

DON'T CARRY A STASH, PUT IT IN THE TRASH.

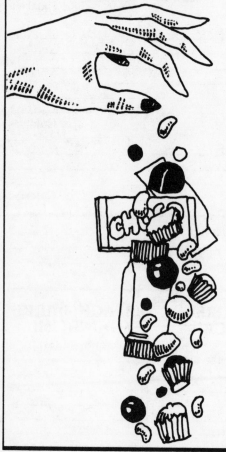

DAY 41

TODAY'S DATE [　　　] TODAY'S WEIGHT [　　　]

BREAKFAST _____
_____
_____
_____ ____ Calories

LUNCH _____
_____
_____
_____
_____ ____ Calories

DINNER _____
_____
_____
_____
_____
_____
_____ ____ Calories

SNACKS _____
_____
_____
_____ ____ Calories

EXERCISES _____
_____
_____
_____

FEATHERS IN MY CAP
(Triumphs Over Temptation)
_____
_____
_____
_____
_____

BLACK MARKS AGAINST ME
(Secret Splurges)
_____
_____
_____
_____
_____

MY DIET DIARY

The Big Lie: "If you don't eat you'll disappear."

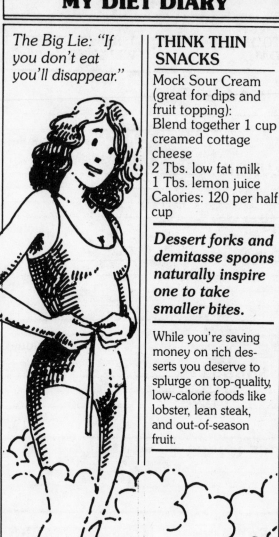

THINK THIN SNACKS

Mock Sour Cream (great for dips and fruit topping):
Blend together 1 cup creamed cottage cheese
2 Tbs. low fat milk
1 Tbs. lemon juice
Calories: 120 per half cup

Dessert forks and demitasse spoons naturally inspire one to take smaller bites.

While you're saving money on rich desserts you deserve to splurge on top-quality, low-calorie foods like lobster, lean steak, and out-of-season fruit.

DAY 42

TODAY'S DATE [   ]   TODAY'S WEIGHT [   ]

BREAKFAST _____
_____
_____
_____ Calories

LUNCH _____
_____
_____
_____
_____ Calories

DINNER _____
_____
_____
_____
_____
_____
_____ Calories

SNACKS _____
_____
_____
_____ Calories

EXERCISES _____
_____
_____
_____

FEATHERS IN MY CAP
(Triumphs Over Temptation)
_____
_____
_____
_____

BLACK MARKS AGAINST ME
(Secret Splurges)
_____
_____
_____
_____

MY DIET DIARY

IF YOU WANT TO FLY WITH THE ANGELS —LIGHTEN UP.

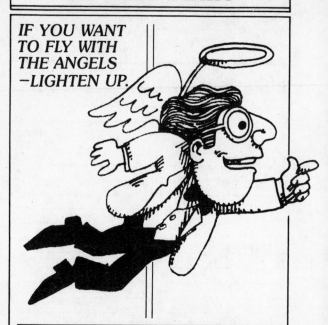

CHEW FOOD SLOWLY: *20 × PER BITE*

THINK THIN SNACKS

Spice up your tuna and cottage cheese with a little horse-radish.

REWARDS

You'll have less weight to tote around with you all the time. The load you carry will be lighter.

For men, being overweight is a potential cause of impotence.

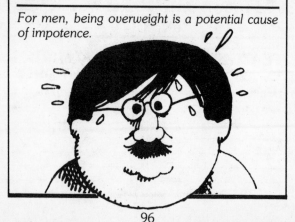

DAY 43

TODAY'S DATE [ ]　　**TODAY'S WEIGHT** [ ]

BREAKFAST _____
_____
_____
_____ Calories

LUNCH _____
_____
_____
_____ Calories

DINNER _____
_____
_____
_____
_____
_____ Calories

SNACKS _____
_____
_____
_____ Calories

EXERCISES _____
_____
_____

FEATHERS IN MY CAP
(Triumphs Over Temptation)
_____
_____
_____
_____

BLACK MARKS AGAINST ME
(Secret Splurges)
_____
_____
_____
_____

97

MY DIET DIARY

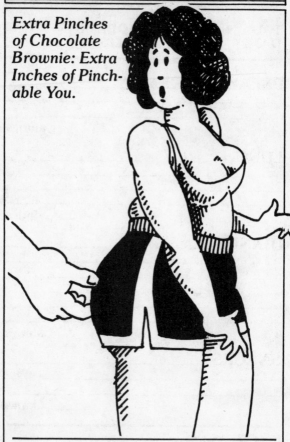

Extra Pinches of Chocolate Brownie: Extra Inches of Pinchable You.

At work, don't eat at your desk. If you have to, borrow someone else's office. You mustn't associate your work space with food.

SMALLER PORTIONS ALWAYS MEANS FEWER CALORIES.

A shot (1½ oz.) of hard liquor (90 proof), be it scotch, gin, rum or whisky has 110 calories, any way you cut it.

Get calorie-free flavor from flavor extracts. A drop of "sherry," "almond," or "pistachio" is a beautiful embellishment on skim milk.

DAY 44

TODAY'S DATE		TODAY'S WEIGHT	

BREAKFAST _____

_____

_____ ____ Calories

LUNCH _____

_____

_____

_____ ____ Calories

DINNER _____

_____

_____

_____

_____

_____ ____ Calories

SNACKS _____

_____

_____ ____ Calories

EXERCISES _____

_____

_____

_____

FEATHERS IN MY CAP (Triumphs Over Temptation)	**BLACK MARKS AGAINST ME** (Secret Splurges)
_____	_____
_____	_____
_____	_____
_____	_____

MY DIET DIARY

YOU CAN BE ANY WEIGHT YOU WANT—IT'S YOUR CHOICE.

Call up the Reserves! Force your body to draw energy from its stored fat instead of from new food.

Imitation cream products (made with vegetable oils) may be lower in cholesterol, but not in calories—and certainly not in artificial chemicals.

PEOPLE LOVE YOU FOR YOUR QUALITIES, NOT YOUR QUANTITIES.

The body is not a garbage truck; don't shovel leftovers into it.

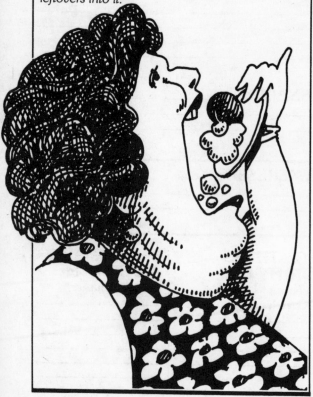

DAY 45

TODAY'S DATE [　　　]   **TODAY'S WEIGHT** [　　　]

BREAKFAST _____
_____
_____
_____ Calories

LUNCH _____
_____
_____
_____
_____ Calories

DINNER _____
_____
_____
_____
_____
_____
_____ Calories

SNACKS _____
_____
_____
_____ Calories

EXERCISES _____
_____
_____
_____

FEATHERS IN MY CAP
(Triumphs Over Temptation)
_____
_____
_____
_____

BLACK MARKS AGAINST ME
(Secret Splurges)
_____
_____
_____
_____

MY DIET DIARY

THINK THIN SNACKS

Pizza????? Yes! As long as you limit it to one 5½-inch slice of a 13¾-inch pie, it's only 155 calories.

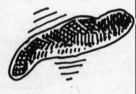

Too much exercise all at once can leave you famished. Exercise moderation in all your activities.

Even the most mundane meal is special when it's served on fine china and crystal goblets.

For every chocolate chip cookie you eat, run five minutes and you won't gain weight. Or don't eat the chocolate chip cookie, run anyway, and lose weight.

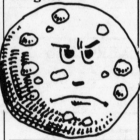

Flavor your rice with soy sauce or tamari instead of high-calorie butter.

REWARDS

The odds are you'll live longer.

DAY 46

TODAY'S DATE [____]   **TODAY'S WEIGHT** [____]

BREAKFAST _____
_____
_____
_____ Calories

LUNCH _____
_____
_____
_____
_____ Calories

DINNER _____
_____
_____
_____
_____
_____
_____ Calories

SNACKS _____
_____
_____
_____ Calories

EXERCISES _____
_____
_____
_____

FEATHERS IN MY CAP
(Triumphs Over Temptation)
_____
_____
_____
_____
_____

BLACK MARKS AGAINST ME
(Secret Splurges)
_____
_____
_____
_____
_____

MY DIET DIARY

Instant and par-boiled rice has 35 calories less per cup than long-cooking rice.

Two slices of bacon are as fattening as one egg.

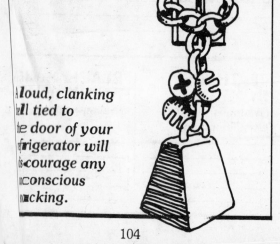

REWARDS
Less weight in your car, more miles to the gallon.

The lighter your eating habits, the more energy you'll have.

A *loud, clanking bell tied to the door of your refrigerator will discourage any unconscious snacking.*

DAY 47

TODAY'S DATE		TODAY'S WEIGHT	

BREAKFAST _____
_____
_____
_____ Calories

LUNCH _____
_____
_____
_____
_____ Calories

DINNER _____
_____
_____
_____
_____
_____ Calories

SNACKS _____
_____
_____
_____ Calories

EXERCISES _____
_____
_____
_____

FEATHERS IN MY CAP
(Triumphs Over Temptation)
_____
_____
_____
_____

BLACK MARKS AGAINST ME
(Secret Splurges)
_____
_____
_____
_____

MY DIET DIARY

REWARDS

More elbow room in the back of Volkswagens.

You'll gain less weight eating 1,500 calories distributed over three meals, than if you eat the same 1,500 calories in one sitting.

Spices add lots of flavor but no calories. Experiment with exotic Indian curries and Chinese pepper blends.

THINK THIN SNACKS

Sprinkle vege-sal seasoning on thin zucchini and carrot wedges.

Broil your fish in white wine instead of butter. The alcohol burns off, leaving no calories but plenty of flavor.

Sharing the responsibility for food preparation with your spouse or children cuts down on your exposure to food.

Think positive thoughts. Berating yourself for being fat only reinforces your fatdom.

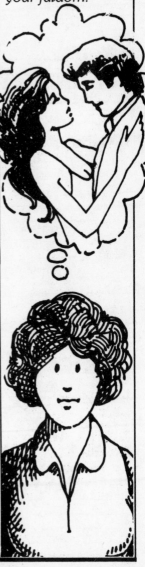

DAY 48

TODAY'S DATE [ ]   **TODAY'S WEIGHT** [ ]

BREAKFAST _____
_____
_____
_____ Calories

LUNCH _____
_____
_____
_____
_____ Calories

DINNER _____
_____
_____
_____
_____
_____ Calories

SNACKS _____
_____
_____
_____ Calories

EXERCISES _____
_____
_____
_____

FEATHERS IN MY CAP
(Triumphs Over Temptation)
_____
_____
_____
_____

BLACK MARKS AGAINST ME
(Secret Splurges)
_____
_____
_____
_____

MY DIET DIARY

VITAMINS ARE FOOD SUPPLE-MENTS, NOT SUBSTITUTES.

Do all your eating in one, specific part of the house. That way you won't associate any other area (TV, the bed, your desk) with food.

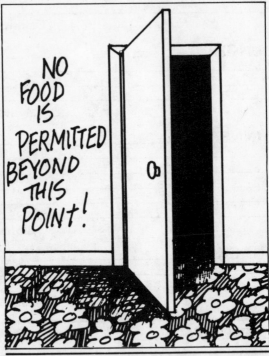

Cream cheese has half the calories of butter. Spread that around.

REWARDS

With a lightened load, your feet will feel better.

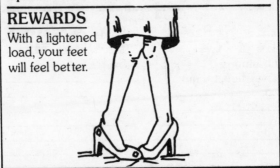

DAY 49

TODAY'S DATE [ ]   **TODAY'S WEIGHT** [ ]

BREAKFAST _____

___ Calories

LUNCH _____

___ Calories

DINNER _____

___ Calories

SNACKS _____

___ Calories

EXERCISES _____

FEATHERS IN MY CAP
(Triumphs Over Temptation)

BLACK MARKS AGAINST ME
(Secret Splurges)

THINK THIN SNACKS

Mix No-Cal chocolate soda and ⅓ cup skim milk for a fat-free ice cream soda without the ice cream. Calories: 22.

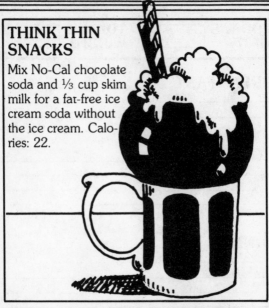

Add hours to your day: If you don't eat right before going to bed, you'll require less sleep.

THINK THIN SNACKS

Chopped scallions or chives add color and flavor to low-fat cottage cheese.

Be your own boss: Don't give in when friends ask you to just try a little dessert.

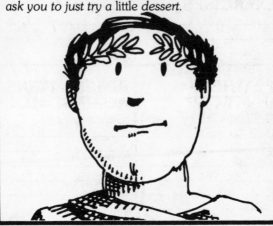

DAY 50

TODAY'S DATE [   ]   **TODAY'S WEIGHT** [   ]

BREAKFAST _____
_____
_____
_____ ____ Calories

LUNCH _____
_____
_____
_____
_____ ____ Calories

DINNER _____
_____
_____
_____
_____
_____
_____ ____ Calories

SNACKS _____
_____
_____
_____ ____ Calories

EXERCISES _____
_____
_____
_____

FEATHERS IN MY CAP
(Triumphs Over Temptation)
_____
_____
_____
_____

BLACK MARKS AGAINST ME
(Secret Splurges)
_____
_____
_____
_____

MY DIET DIARY

Mix your drinks with water or plain soda. Tonic adds **88** calories per 8-ounce glass; bitter lemon adds **125**.

DON'T CONFUSE FOOD HUNGER WITH EMOTIONAL HUNGER.

Instead of thinking about the foods you can't eat, think about the wonderful low-calorie meals you can eat.

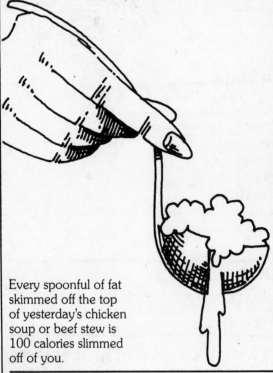

Every spoonful of fat skimmed off the top of yesterday's chicken soup or beef stew is 100 calories slimmed off of you.

Take off two-thirds of a pound every week simply by jogging for half an hour daily—that comes to 34 pounds a year!

Alcohol: The lower the spirit, the lower the calories. One hundred-proof liquors average **83** calories per ounce. Eighty-proof average **63**.

DAY 51

TODID'S DATE [   ]   TODAY'S WEIGHT [   ]

BREAKFAST _____
_____
_____
_____ Calories

LUNCH _____
_____
_____
_____
_____ Calories

DINNER _____
_____
_____
_____
_____
_____ Calories

SNACKS _____
_____
_____
_____ Calories

EXERCISES _____
_____
_____
_____

FEATHERS IN MY CAP
(Triumphs Over Temptation)
_____
_____
_____
_____
_____

BLACK MARKS AGAINST ME
(Secret Splurges)
_____
_____
_____
_____
_____

113

MY DIET DIARY

Buttermilk has half the calories of whole milk and is great for thickening gravies and sauces.

An occasional trip to the local health club (many accept single-admission visitors) is a great inspiration to get into shape. It may lead to regular workouts.

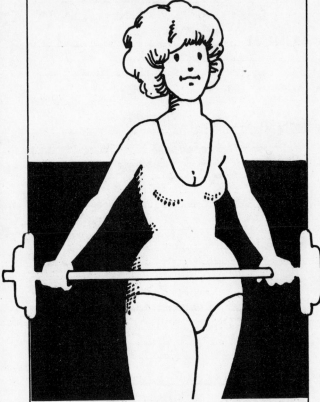

A cup of creamed chipped beef is only 35 calories more than a cup of dried chipped beef.

A glass of tomato juice has half the calories of orange or grapefruit juice, and it's more filling.

Eight ounces of chocolate milk has 115 more calories than 8 ounces of skim.

DAY 52

TODAY'S DATE [　　] **TODAY'S WEIGHT** [　　]

BREAKFAST _____
_____
_____
_____ Calories

LUNCH _____
_____
_____
_____
_____ Calories

DINNER _____
_____
_____
_____
_____
_____
_____ Calories

SNACKS _____
_____
_____
_____ Calories

EXERCISES _____
_____
_____
_____

FEATHERS IN MY CAP
(Triumphs Over Temptation)
_____
_____
_____
_____
_____

BLACK MARKS AGAINST ME
(Secret Splurges)
_____
_____
_____
_____
_____

MY DIET DIARY

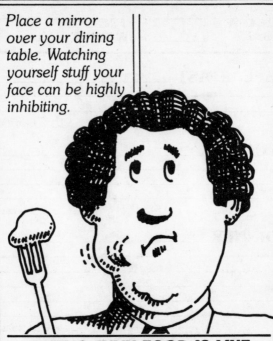

Place a mirror over your dining table. Watching yourself stuff your face can be highly inhibiting.

EATING JUNK FOOD IS LIKE LITTERING YOUR BODY.

At 65 calories per tablespoon, honey is no substitute for sugar, which has 45 calories per tablespoon.

Losing only a pound or two a week gives the dieter time to adjust to his or her new, thinner image.

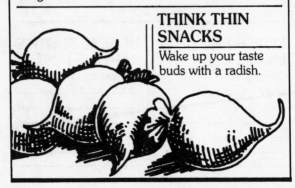

THINK THIN SNACKS

Wake up your taste buds with a radish.

DAY 53

TODAY'S DATE [ ] **TODAY'S WEIGHT** [ ]

BREAKFAST _____
_____
_____
_____ ____ Calories

LUNCH _____
_____
_____
_____
_____ ____ Calories

DINNER _____
_____
_____
_____
_____
_____
_____ ____ Calories

SNACKS _____
_____
_____
_____ ____ Calories

EXERCISES _____
_____
_____
_____

FEATHERS IN MY CAP
(Triumphs Over Temptation)
_____
_____
_____
_____
_____

BLACK MARKS AGAINST ME
(Secret Splurges)
_____
_____
_____
_____
_____

117

MY DIET DIARY

Eating burns 90 calories an hour, but eating for an hour can add thousands of calories.

Creating fullness: Close your eyes and think about how your stomach feels when it is full. Imagine that bloated sensation. Feel that you just finished a five-course meal and you can't stomach another bite.

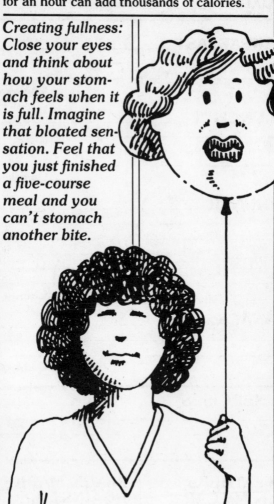

Store fattening foods (if you must keep them in the refrigerator) in opaque containers. Store skinny snacks in see-through cellophane.

THINNESS AND SELF CONTROL HAVE A LOT IN COMMON.

DAY 54

TODAY'S DATE		TODAY'S WEIGHT	

BREAKFAST _____
_____
_____
_____ ____ Calories

LUNCH _____
_____
_____
_____
_____ ____ Calories

DINNER _____
_____
_____
_____
_____
_____
_____ ____ Calories

SNACKS _____
_____
_____
_____ ____ Calories

EXERCISES _____
_____
_____
_____

FEATHERS IN MY CAP (Triumphs Over Temptation)	**BLACK MARKS AGAINST ME** (Secret Splurges)
_____	_____
_____	_____
_____	_____
_____	_____

MY DIET DIARY

A 4-ounce glass of dry table wine has 64 calories less than sweet dessert wine.

At large parties and picnic-style barbeques no one will notice how little you are eating.

3,500 CALORIES = APPROXIMATELY ONE POUND OF BODY WEIGHT.

All calories are created equal—be they from cake or from meat—but some calories are more nutritious than others.

Climbing the stairs instead of taking the escalator saves time and tones legs.

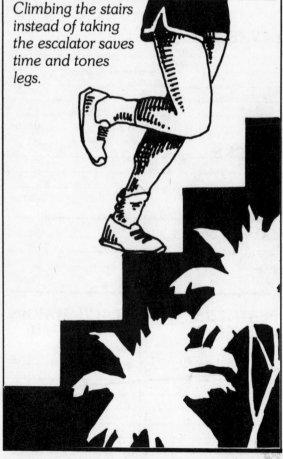

DAY 55

TODAY'S DATE [ ]   **TODAY'S WEIGHT** [ ]

BREAKFAST _____
_____
_____
_____ Calories

LUNCH _____
_____
_____
_____ Calories

DINNER _____
_____
_____
_____
_____
_____ Calories

SNACKS _____
_____
_____
_____ Calories

EXERCISES _____
_____
_____
_____

FEATHERS IN MY CAP
(Triumphs Over Temptation)
_____
_____
_____
_____

BLACK MARKS AGAINST ME
(Secret Splurges)
_____
_____
_____
_____

121

MY DIET DIARY

The hotter the potato, the more absorbent it is. Let it cool and use less butter.

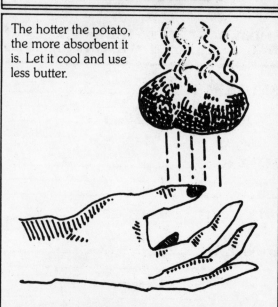

TAKE THE TIME TO TASTE WHAT YOU'RE EATING.

Whole milk has almost twice the calories of skim—and skim is easier to digest.

Instead of getting a donut, call up a friend during your coffee break.

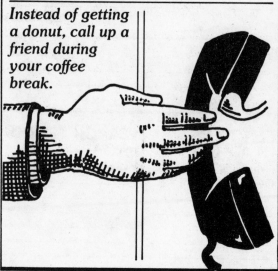

DAY 56

TODAY'S DATE [ ] **TODAY'S WEIGHT** [ ]

BREAKFAST _____
_____
_____
_____ Calories

LUNCH _____
_____
_____
_____
_____ Calories

DINNER _____
_____
_____
_____
_____
_____
_____ Calories

SNACKS _____
_____
_____
_____ Calories

EXERCISES _____
_____
_____

FEATHERS IN MY CAP
(Triumphs Over Temptation)

BLACK MARKS AGAINST ME
(Secret Splurges)

MY DIET DIARY

Calories do count; don't squander them on food you don't really enjoy.

THINK THIN SNACKS

Thicken up bouillon with sliced mushrooms, bean sprouts, or minced carrots—they take only about two minutes to cook in the broth.

Willpower is developed gradually, like a muscle, by daily exercise.

THE BEST WAY TO DIET IS TO KEEP YOUR MOUTH SHUT.

Create a feeling of fullness before meals with a glass of low-calorie vegetable juice or a small bowl of salad greens.

If you put your fork down between bites, you can't "shovel" your food.

Just because you went off your diet for a little while is no excuse to stay off it.

Slow down for a mid-afternoon cup of herbal tea. Your body will thank you.

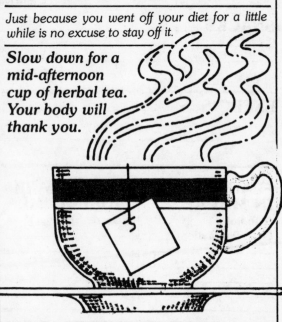

DAY 57

TODAY'S DATE [ ]   **TODAY'S WEIGHT** [ ]

BREAKFAST _____
_____
_____
_____ Calories

LUNCH _____
_____
_____
_____
_____ Calories

DINNER _____
_____
_____
_____
_____
_____
_____ Calories

SNACKS _____
_____
_____
_____ Calories

EXERCISES _____
_____
_____
_____

FEATHERS IN MY CAP
(Triumphs Over Temptation)
_____
_____
_____
_____

BLACK MARKS AGAINST ME
(Secret Splurges)
_____
_____
_____
_____

MY DIET DIARY

If you really like to eat so much, give yourself the time to taste each bite; don't wolf it down.

LET YOUR FOOD BE HIGH IN QUALITY, NOT QUANTITY.

A half-hour of brisk walking burns up 300 calories and gives a glow to the body, mind and spirit.

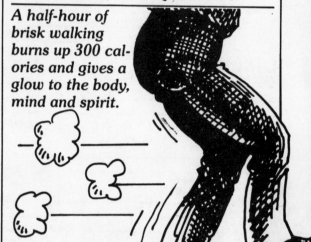

ONCE YOU'VE HAD A TASTE, YOU'VE EXPERIENCED IT ALL.

Treat yourself to a fresh supply of herbs and spices. You deserve all the flavor you can get.

Your appearance speaks loudly of how you feel about yourself.

THINK THIN SNACKS

Lettuce or cabbage leaves, zucchini or cucumber slabs, and thick slices of apple or pineapple can "sandwich" a spread just as well as bread.

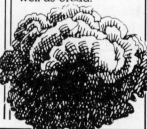

DAY 58

TODAY'S DATE [   ]   **TODAY'S WEIGHT** [   ]

BREAKFAST _____
_____
_____
_____ ___ Calories

LUNCH _____
_____
_____
_____
_____ ___ Calories

DINNER _____
_____
_____
_____
_____
_____
_____ ___ Calories

SNACKS _____
_____
_____
_____ ___ Calories

EXERCISES _____
_____
_____
_____

FEATHERS IN MY CAP
(Triumphs Over Temptation)
_____
_____
_____
_____

BLACK MARKS AGAINST ME
(Secret Splurges)
_____
_____
_____
_____

MY DIET DIARY

OLD ADAGE: NEVER TOO RICH; NEVER TOO THIN.

Six ounces of tonic water has 71 calories more than 6 ounces of plain seltzer. They are *not* interchangeable.

Arrange to meet business associates in their offices instead of in restaurants.

STICK TO YOUR DIET TODAY. YOU'LL FEEL BETTER ABOUT YOURSELF TOMORROW.

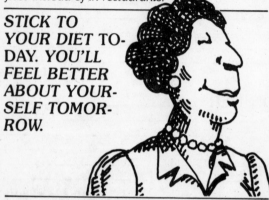

Both spring water and tap water have zero calories, but spring water tastes better.

AT A BUFFET, YOU DON'T HAVE TO SAMPLE EVERYTHING.

REWARDS
Feeling more energetic

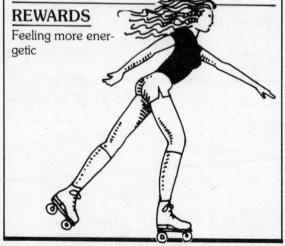

DAY 59

TODAY'S DATE		TODAY'S WEIGHT	

BREAKFAST _____

_____
_____
_____ Calories

LUNCH _____

_____
_____
_____
_____ Calories

DINNER _____

_____
_____
_____
_____
_____
_____ Calories

SNACKS _____

_____
_____
_____ Calories

EXERCISES _____

_____
_____
_____

FEATHERS IN MY CAP (Triumphs Over Temptation)	**BLACK MARKS AGAINST ME** (Secret Splurges)
_____	_____
_____	_____
_____	_____
_____	_____

MY DIET DIARY

REWARDS
No more unsightly bulges.

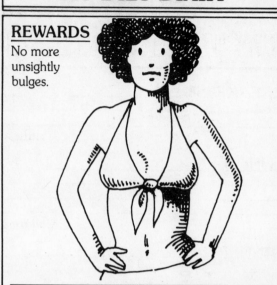

You can have two 5-ounce glasses of table wine for the same number of calories as one mixed cocktail or a 12-ounce can of beer.

LONG-TERM RESULTS CALL FOR LONG-TERM EFFORTS.

THINK THIN SNACKS
A drop of saccharin on the tip of the tongue can take the place of a mound of candy.

Go to bed with an empty stomach and promise yourself a delicious breakfast the next morning.

Remove from the table all the food that you don't plan to eat.

Restless? Don't run to your refrigerator—run around the block instead.

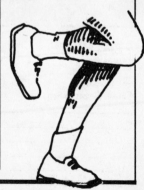

DAY 60

TODAY'S DATE		TODAY'S WEIGHT	

BREAKFAST _____
_____
_____
_____ ____ Calories

LUNCH _____
_____
_____
_____
_____ ____ Calories

DINNER _____
_____
_____
_____
_____
_____
_____ ____ Calories

SNACKS _____
_____
_____
_____ ____ Calories

EXERCISES _____
_____
_____

FEATHERS IN MY CAP
(Triumphs Over Temptation)
_____
_____
_____
_____

BLACK MARKS AGAINST ME
(Secret Splurges)
_____
_____
_____
_____
_____

131

60-DAY WEIGHT CHART

DAY		DAY	
1	_____	31	_____
2	_____	32	_____
3	_____	33	_____
4	_____	34	_____
5	_____	35	_____
6	_____	36	_____
7	_____	37	_____
8	_____	38	_____
9	_____	39	_____
10	_____	40	_____
11	_____	41	_____
12	_____	42	_____
13	_____	43	_____
14	_____	44	_____
15	_____	45	_____
16	_____	46	_____
17	_____	47	_____
18	_____	48	_____
19	_____	49	_____
20	_____	50	_____
21	_____	51	_____
22	_____	52	_____
23	_____	53	_____
24	_____	54	_____
25	_____	55	_____
26	_____	56	_____
27	_____	57	_____
28	_____	58	_____
29	_____	59	_____
30	_____	60	_____

FULL LENGTH PHOTO
DAY 60

*Bust/Chest*_____

*Waist*_____

*Hips*_____

DIET DIARY WEIGHT AND CALORIE TABLE COUNTER

SUGGESTED BODY WEIGHTS
Range of Acceptable Weight

Height (Feet-inches)	Men (Pounds)	Women (Pounds)
4'10"		92–119
4'11"		94–122
5'0"		96–125
5'1"		99–128
5'2"	112–141	102–131
5'3"	115–144	105–134
5'4"	118–148	108–138
5'5"	121–152	111–142
5'6"	124–156	114–146
5'7"	128–161	118–150
5'8"	132–166	122–154
5'9"	136–170	126–158
5'10"	140–174	130–163
5'11"	144–179	134–168
6'0"	148–184	138–173
6'1"	152–189	
6'2"	156–194	
6'3"	160–199	
6'4"	164–204	

NOTE: Height without shoes; weight without clothes.
SOURCE: Fogarty Conference on Obesity, 1973.

The table of acceptable weight ranges for adults can help you estimate how much weight you need to lose. If you have a small frame, your ideal weight probably is at the low end of the range; if medium, at the middle; if large, at the high end of the range.

Remember—the weight that is best for you in your mid-twenties is best for you in later years, too.

CALORIE TABLES
Calorie values given for foods in the following tables do not include calories from added fat, sugar, sauce, or dressing—unless such items are included in the listing. Cup measure refers to a standard 8-ounce measuring cup, unless otherwise stated.

BEVERAGES
Not including milk and fruit juices

Alcoholic beverages	Calories
Beer, 3.6% alcohol, *8-ounce glass*	100
12-ounce can or bottle	150
Whiskey, gin, rum, vodka	
80-proof, 1½-ounce jigger	95
86-proof, 1½-ounce jigger	105
90-proof, 1½-ounce jigger	110
100-proof, 1½-ounce jigger	125
Wines, table (Chablis, claret, Rhine wine, sauterne, etc.), *3½-ounce glass*	85
Wines, dessert (muscatel, port, sherry, Tokay, etc.), *3½-ounce glass*	140

Carbonated beverages	Calories
Cola-type, *8-ounce glass*	95
12-ounce can or bottle	145
Fruit flavors, 10–13% sugar	
8-ounce glass	115
12-ounce can or bottle	170

Ginger ale, *8-ounce glass*	**75**
12-ounce can or bottle	**115**
Root beer, *8-ounce glass*	**100**
12-ounce can or bottle	**150**

BREADS AND CEREALS

Bread	Calories
Cracked wheat, 18 slices per pound loaf, *1 slice*	**65**
Raisin, 18 slices per pound loaf, *1 slice*	**65**
Rye, 18 slices per pound loaf, *1 slice*	**56**
White	
soft crumb	
regular slice, 18 slices per pound loaf, *1 slice*	**70**
thin slice, 22 slices per pound loaf, *1 slice*	**55**
firm crumb, 20 slices per pound loaf, *1 slice*	**65**
Whole wheat	
soft crumb, 16 slices per pound loaf, *1 slice*	**65**
firm crumb, 18 slices per pound loaf, *1 slice*	**60**

Breakfast cereals	Calories
Bran flakes	
(40% bran) *1 ounce (about 4/5 cup)*	**85**
with raisins, *1 ounce (about 3/5 cup)*	**80**
Corn	
puffed, presweetened, *1 ounce (about 1 cup)*	**115**
shredded, *1 ounce (about 1-1/6 cups)*	**110**
Corn flakes	
plain, *1 ounce (about 1-1/6 cups)*	**110**
sugar-coated, *1 ounce (about ⅔ cup)*	**110**
Farina, cooked, quick-cooking, *¾ cup*	**80**
Oats, puffed	
plain, *1 ounce (about 1-1/6 cups)*	**115**
sugar-coated, *1 ounce (about 4/5 cup)*	**115**
Oatmeal or rolled oats, cooked, *¾ cup*	**100**
Rice	
flakes, *1 ounce (about 1 cup)*	**110**
puffed, *1 ounce (about 2 cups)*	**115**
pre-sweetened, *1 ounce (about ⅔ cup)*	**110**
shredded, *1 ounce (about 1⅛ cups*	**115**
Wheat	
puffed, *1 ounce (about 1⅞ cups)*	**105**
puffed, pre-sweetened, *1 ounce (about 4/5 cup)*	**105**
rolled, cooked, *¾ cup*	**135**
shredded, plain, *1 ounce (1 large biscuit or ½ cup bite-size)*	**100**
flakes, *1 ounce (about 1 cup)*	**100**

Other grain products	Calories
Corn grits, degermed, cooked, *¾ cup*	**95**
Macaroni, cooked	
plain, *¾ cup*	**115**
with cheese	
home recipe, *½ cup*	**215**
canned, *½ cup*	**115**
Noodles, cooked, *¾ cup*	**150**
Rice, cooked, instant, *¾ cup*	**135**
Spaghetti, cooked	
plain, *¾ cup*	**115**
in tomato sauce, with cheese, home recipe, *¾ cup*	**195**

in tomato sauce, with cheese, canned, ¾ *cup*	140
with meatballs, home recipe, ¾ *cup*	250
with meatballs, canned, ¾ *cup*	195
Wheat germ, toasted, *1 tablespoon*	25

Other flour-based foods	Calories

Cakes, cookies, pies—See Desserts.
Cracker

butter, about *2-inch diameter, one*	15
cheese, about *2-inch diameter, one*	15
graham, *2½-inches square, two*	55
matzo, *6-inch diameter piece, one*	80
oyster, *ten*	35
pilot, *one*	75
rye, *1⅞ x 3½-inches, two*	45
saltines, *1⅞-inches square, four*	50

Doughnut

Cake-type, plain, *3¼-inch diameter (1½ ounces) one*	165
Yeast-leaven, raised, *3¾-inch diameter (1½ ounces) one*	175
Danish pastry, plain, *4½-inch diameter, one*	275

Pancake (griddle cakes)

Wheat (home recipe or mix), *4-inch cake, one one*	60
Buckwheat (mix), *4-inch cake, one*	55

Pizza, plain cheese, *5⅓-inch sector of 13¾-inch pie* — 155

Pretzel

Dutch, twisted, *one*	60
Stick, *5 regular (3⅛-inches long)* or *10 small (2¼-inches long)*	10

Spoonbread, ½ cup	235
Waffle, *7 inch*	210

DESSERTS AND OTHER SWEETS

Cakes	Calories
Angelcake, *2½-inch sector of 9¾-inch round cake*	135
Boston cream pie, *2⅛-inch sector of 8-inch round cake*	210
Chocolate cake, with chocolate icing, *1¾-inch sector of 9-inch round layer cake*	235
Fruitcake, dark, *2 × 1½ × ¼-inch slice*	55
Gingerbread, *2¾ × 2¾ × 1⅜-inch slice*	175

Plain cake

without icing	
3 × 3 × 2-inch slice	315
2¾-inch diameter cupcake	115
with chocolate icing	
1¾-inch sector of 9-inch round layer cake	240
2¾-inch diameter cupcake	170

Pound cake, old fashion, *3½ × 3 × ½-inch slice*	140
Sponge cake, *1⅞-inch sector of 9¾-inch round cake*	145

Candies	Calories
Caramels *(1 ounce) 3 medium*	115
Chocolate creams, 35 to a pound, *2 to 3 pieces (1 ounce)*	125

Chocolate, milk, sweetened, *1-ounce bar* — 145
Chocolate, milk, sweetened, with almonds,
   1-ounce bar — 150
Chocolate mints, 20 to a pound, *1 to 2 mints*
   (1 ounce) — 115
Fondant
   candy corn, *20 pieces (1 ounce)* — 105
   mints, *three 1½-inch mints (1 ounce)* — 105
Fudge, vanilla or chocolate
   plain
      1 ounce — 115
      1-inch cube — 85
   with nuts
      1 ounce — 120
      1-inch cube — 90
Gumdrops, about *2½ large or 20 small*
   (1 ounce) — 100
Hard candy, *three or four ¾-inch-diameter*
   candy balls (1 ounce) — 110
Jellybeans, *10 (1 ounce)* — 105
Marshmallows, *4 large* — 90
Peanut brittle, *1½ pieces, 2½ × 1¼ × ⅜-inch*
   (1 ounce) — 120

Other sweets	Calories
Chocolate	
bittersweet, *1-ounce square*	135
semisweet, *1-ounce square*	145
Chocolate syrup	
thin type, *1 tablespoon*	45
fudge type, *1 tablespoon*	60
Cranberry sauce, canned, *1 tablespoon*	25
Honey, *1 tablespoon*	65
Jam, preserves, *1 tablespoon*	55
Jelly, marmalade, *1 tablespoon*	50
Molasses, *1 tablespoon*	50
Syrup, table blends, *1 tablespoon*	55
Sugar, white, granulated, or brown (packed), *1 teaspoon*	15

Cookies	Calories
Chocolate chip, *2⅓-inch cooky, ½-inch thick*	50
Figbar, *1 small*	50
Sandwich, chocolate or vanilla, *1¾-inch cooky, ⅜-inch thick*	50
Vanilla wafer, *1¾-inch cooky*	20

Pies	Calories
Apple, *⅛ of 9-inch pie*	300
Blueberry, *⅛ of 9-inch pie*	285
Cherry, *⅛ of 9-inch pie*	310
Chocolate meringue, *⅛ of 9-inch pie*	285
Coconut custard, *⅛ of 9-inch pie*	270
Custard, plain, *⅛ of 9-inch pie*	250
Lemon meringue, *⅛ of 9-inch pie*	270
Mince, *⅛ of 9-inch pie*	320
Peach, *⅛ of 9-inch pie*	300
Pecan, *⅛ of 9-inch pie*	430
Pumpkin, *⅛ of 9-inch pie*	240
Raisin, *⅛ of 9-inch pie*	320
Rhubarb, *⅛ of 9-inch pie*	300
Strawberry, *⅛ of 9-inch pie*	185

Other desserts	Calories
Apple betty, ½ cup	160
Bread pudding, with raisins, ½ cup	250
Brownie, with nuts, 1¾-inches square, ⅞-inch thick	90
Custard, baked, ½ cup	150
Fruit ice, ½ cup	125

FATS, OILS, CREAMS AND RELATED PRODUCTS

Fats and oils	Calories
Butter or margarine	
1 pat, 1-inch square, ⅓-inch thick,	35
1 tablespoon	100
Margarine, whipped, soft, tub, 1 tablespoon	100
Cooking fats	
vegetable, 1 tablespoon	110
lard, 1 tablespoon	115
Peanut butter, see Meats, Poultry, Fish, Eggs, Dried Beans and Peas, and Nuts	
Salad dressings	
regular	
blue cheese, 1 tablespoon	75
French, 1 tablespoon	65
home-cooked, boiled, 1 tablespoon	25
Italian, 1 tablespoon	70
mayonnaise, 1 tablespoon	100
salad dressing, commercial, plain (mayonnaise-type), 1 tablespoon	55
Russian, 1 tablespoon	75
Thousand Island, 1 tablespoon	60
low calorie	
French, 1 tablespoon	20
Italian, 1 tablespoon	15
Thousand Island, 1 tablespoon	25
Salad oil, 1 tablespoon	120

Cream	Calories
half-and-half (milk and cream)	
1 tablespoon	20
1 cup	315
Light, coffee or table, 1 tablespoon	30
Sour, 1 tablespoon	25
Whipped topping, pressurized, 1 tablespoon	10
Whipping	
heavy, 1 tablespoon	50
light, 1 tablespoon	45

MEAT, POULTRY, FISH, EGGS, DRIED BEANS AND PEAS, AND NUTS

Beef and Veal	Calories
Beef and vegetable stew	
canned, 1 cup	195
homemade, with lean beef, 1 cup	220
Beef pot pie, home prepared, baked, ¼ of 9-inch diameter pie	385
Chili con carne, canned	
without beans, ½ cup	240
with beans, ½ cup	170
Corned beef, canned, 3 ounces	185
Corned beef hash, 2/5 cup (3 ounces)	155

Dried beef
chipped, ⅓ cup (2 ounces)	115
creamed, ½ cup	190

Hamburger, broiled, panbroiled, or sauteed
regular, 3 ounces	245
lean, 3 ounces	185

Oven roast, cooked, without bone
cuts relatively fat, such as rib
lean and fat, 3 ounces	375
lean only, 3 ounces	205

cuts relatively lean, such as round
lean and fat, 3 ounces	220
lean only, 3 ounces	160

Pot roast, cooked, braised or simmered, without bone
lean and fat, 3 ounces	245
lean only, 3 ounces	165

Steak, broiled, without bone
cuts relatively fat, such as sirloin
lean and fat, 3 ounces	330
lean only, 3 ounces	175

cuts relatively lean, such as round
lean and fat, 3 ounces	220
lean only, 3 ounces	160

Veal cutlet, broiled, without bone, trimmed, 3 ounces — 185
Veal roast, cooked, without bone, 3 ounces — 230

Lamb — Calories

Loin chop, broiled, without bone
lean and fat, 3 ounces	305
lean only, 3 ounces	160

Leg, roasted, without bone
lean and fat, 3 ounces	235
lean only, 3 ounces	160

Shoulder, roasted, without bone
lean and fat, 3 ounces	285
lean only, 3 ounces	175

Pork — Calories

Bacon, broiled or fried, crisp
2 thin slices	60
2 medium slices	85

Bacon, Canadian, cooked, one 3⅜ × 3/16-inch slice — 60

Chop, broiled without bone
lean and fat, 3 ounces	335
lean only, 3 ounces	230

Ham, cured, cooked, without bone
lean and fat, 3 ounces	245
lean only, 3 ounces	160

Roast, loin, cooked, without bone
lean and fat, 3 ounces	310
lean only, 3 ounces	215

Poultry — Calories

Chicken
roasted (no skin) breast, one-half	140

fried (no skin)
breast, one-half	160
thigh, one	115
drumstick, one	80
canned, meat with broth, ½ cup (3½ ounces)	165

Poultry pie, home prepared, baked, ¼ of 9-inch diameter pie — 410

Turkey, roasted (no skin)

light meat, *3 ounces*	135
dark meat, *3 ounces*	160

Fish and shellfish Calories

Bluefish, baked, *3 ounces*
(3½ × 2 × ½-inch piece) — 135
Clams, shelled
    canned, *3 medium clams and juice (3 ounces)* — 45
    raw, meat only, *4 medium (3 ounces)* — 65
Crabmeat, canned or cooked, *½ cup (3 ounces)* — 80
Fish sticks, breaded, cooked
    frozen, *three 4 × 1 × ½-inch sticks (3 ounces)* — 150
Haddock, breaded, fried, *3 ounces (4 × 2½ ×*
½-inch fillet) — 140
Mackerel
    broiled with fat, *3 ounces*
    (4 × 3 × ½-inch piece) — 200
    canned, *²/₅ cup with liquid (3 ounces)* — 155
Ocean perch, breaded, fried,
    3 ounces, (4 × 2½ × ½-inch piece) — 195
Oysters, raw, meat only, *½ cup (6 to 10 medium)* — 80
Salmon
    broiled or baked, *3 ounces* — 155
    canned, pink, *³/₅ cup with liquid (3 ounces)* — 120
Sardines, canned in oil, drained, *7 medium (3*
ounces) — 170
Shrimp, canned, *27 medium (3 ounces)* — 100
Tunafish, canned in oil, drained, *½ cup (3*
ounces) — 170

Eggs Calories

Fried in fat, *large, one*	95
Hard or soft cooked, "boiled", *large, one*	80
Omelet, plain, *1 large egg, milk, and fat for cooking*	110
Poached, *large, one*	80
Scrambled in fat, *1 large egg and milk*	110

Dried beans and peas Calories

Baked beans, canned
    with pork and tomato sauce, *½ cup* — 155
    with pork and sweet sauce, *½ cup* — 190
Limas, cooked, *½ cup* — 130

Nuts Calories

Almonds, *15 (2 tablespoons)*	105
Brazil nuts, *4–5 large (2 tablespoons)*	115
Cashews, *11–12 medium (2 tablespoons)*	100
Coconut, fresh, shredded, *2 tablespoons*	55
Peanuts, *2 tablespoons*	105
Peanut butter, *1 tablespoon*	95
Pecans, halves, *10 jumbo or 15 large*	95

Walnuts
    black, chopped, *2 tablespoons* — 100
    English or Persian
        halves, *6 or 7* — 80
        chopped, *2 tablespoons* — 105

MILK AND CHEESE

Milk Calories

Buttermilk, *1 cup*	100
Condensed, *sweetened, undiluted, ½ cup*	490

	Calories
Evaporated, whole, undiluted, ½ cup	170
Lowfat, 2% fat, nonfat milk solids added, *1 cup*	125
Skim, *1 cup*	85
Whole, *1 cup*	150

Yogurt	Calories
Made from skim milk, *1 cup*	125
Made from whole milk, *1 cup*	140

Milk beverages	Calories
Chocolate, homemade, *1 cup*	240
Chocolate milkshake, *one 12-ounce container*	405
Cocoa, homemade, *1 cup*	220
Malted milk, *1 cup*	235

Milk desserts	Calories
Custard, baked, *1 cup*	305
Ice cream	
regular (about 10% fat), *1 cup*	270
rich (about 16% fat), *1 cup*	350
Ice milk	
hardened, *1 cup*	185
soft-serve, *1 cup*	225
Sherbet, ½ cup	135

Cheese	Calories
American	
process	
1 ounce	105
1-inch cube	60
process cheese food	
1 tablespoon	45
1-inch cube	55
process cheese spread *1 tablespoon*	40
1 ounce	80
Blue or roquefort-type	
1 ounce	100
1-inch cube	60
Camembert, *1 wedge of a 4-ounce package*	
containing 3 wedges	115
Cheddar, natural	
1 ounce	115
1-inch cube	70
½ cup, grated (2 ounces)	225
Cottage	
creamed	
2 tablespoons (1 ounce)	30
1 cup, packed	250
uncreamed	
2 tablespoons (1 ounce)	25
1 cup, packed	170
Cream	
1 ounce	100
1-inch cube	55
Parmesan, grated	
1 tablespoon	25
1 ounce	130
Swiss, natural	
1 ounce	105
1-inch cube	55
Swiss, process	
1 ounce	95
1-inch cube	60

SNACKS AND OTHER "EXTRAS"

Bouillon cube, *1 cube, ½ inch*	5
Cheese sauce (medium white sauce with 2 tablespoons grated cheese per cup) *½ cup*	205
Corn chips, *1 cup*	230
Doughnut	
cake-type, plain, *3¼-inch diameter (1½ ounces), one*	165
yeast-leavened, raised, *3¾-inch diameter (1½ ounces), one*	175
French fries	
fresh, *ten 3½ × ¼-inch pieces*	215
frozen, *ten 3½ × ¼-inch pieces*	170
Gravy, *2 tablespoons*	35
Hamburger (with roll), *2-ounce patty*	280
Hot dog (with roll), *1 average*	290
Olives	
green, *5 small or 3 large or 2 giant*	15
ripe, *3 small or 2 large*	15
Pickles	
dill, *1¾ × 4-inch pickle*	15
sweet, *¾ × 2½-inch pickle*	20
Pizza, plain cheese, *5⅓-inch sector of 13¾-inch pie*	155
Popcorn, large-kernel, popped with oil and salt, *1 cup*	40
Potato chips, *ten 1¾ × 2½-inch chips*	115
Pretzel	
Dutch, twisted, *one*	60
stick, *5 regular (3⅛-inches long) or 10 small (2¼-inches long)*	10
Tomato catsup or **chili sauce,** *1 tablespoon*	15
White sauce, medium (1 cup milk, 2 tablespoons fat, 2 tablespoons flour) *½ cup*	200

VEGETABLES AND FRUITS

Good sources of vitamin C are marked (CC), fair sources are marked (C), and good sources of vitamin A are marked (A)

Vegetables (raw):	Calories
Cabbage (C)	
plain, shredded, chopped, or sliced, *½ cup*	10
coleslaw	
with mayonnaise, *½ cup*	85
with mayonnaise-type salad dressing, *½ cup*	60
Carrots (A)	
7½ × 1⅛-inch carrot	30
½ cup, grated	25
Celery, *three 5-inch stalks*	10
Chicory, *½ cup, ½-inch pieces*	5
Chives, *1 tablespoon*	Trace
Cucumbers, pared, *6 center slices, ⅛-inch thick*	5
Endive, *½ cup, small pieces*	5
Lettuce	
leaves, *large, two*	5
shredded or chopped, *½ cup*	5
wedge, *⅙ head, one*	10
Onions	
young green	
chopped, *1 tablespoon*	5
without tops, *2 medium or 6 small*	15
mature	
chopped, *1 tablespoon*	5

Parsley, chopped, *1 tablespoon*	Trace
Peppers, green	
chopped, *1 tablespoon*	Trace
ring, *¼-inch thick, one*	Trace
Radishes, *5 medium*	5
Tomatoes (C), *2 ²/₅-inch diameter tomato, one*	20
Turnips, cubed or sliced, *½ cup*	20
Watercress, *10 sprigs*	5

Vegetables (cooked, canned, or frozen)	Calories
Asparagus spears (C), *6 medium or ½ cup cut*	20
Beans	
green lima, *½ cup*	90
snap, green, wax, or yellow, *½ cup*	15
Beets, diced, sliced, or small whole, *½ cup*	30
Beet greens (A), *½ cup*	15
Broccoli (A, CC)	
chopped, *½ cup*	25
stalks, *4½ to 5-inch*	25
Brussels sprouts (CC), *½ cup (four 1¼ to 1½-inch sprouts)*	25
Cabbage (C), *½ cup*	15
Carrots (A), *½ cup*	25
Cauliflower (C), flower buds, *½ cup*	15
Celery, diced, *½ cup*	10
Chard (A), *½ cup*	15
Collard (A,C), *½ cup*	25
Corn	
on cob, *one 5-inch ear*	70
kernels, drained, *½ cup*	70
cream-style, *½ cup*	105
Cress, garden (A,C), *½ cup*	15
Dandelion greens (A), *½ cup*	15
Eggplant, diced, *½ cup*	20
Kale (A,C), *½ cup*	20
Kohlrabi (C), *½ cup*	20
Mushrooms, canned, *½ cup*	20
Mustard greens (A,C), *½ cup*	15
Okra	
cuts and pods, *½ cup*	35
sliced, *½ cup*	25
Onions, mature, *½ cup*	30
Parsnips	
diced, *½ cup*	50
mashed, *½ cup*	70
Peas, green, *½ cup*	65
Peppers, green (CC), *1 medium*	15
Potatoes	
au gratin, *½ cup*	180
baked (C), *2⅓-inch diameter, 4¾-inch long, one*	145
boiled, *2½-inch diameter whole, one*	90
diced, *½ cup*	55
chips, *ten 1¾ × 2½-inch*	115
french fries	
fresh, *ten 1½ × ¼-inch pieces*	215
frozen, *ten 3½ × ¼-inch pieces*	170
hash-browned, *½ cup*	175
mashed	
milk added, *½ cup*	70
milk and fat added, *½ cup*	100
made from granules with milk and fat added, *½ cup*	100
pan-fried from raw, *½ cup*	230

salad	
made with cooked salad dressing ½ cup	125
made with mayonnaise or French	
dressing and eggs, ½ cup	180
scalloped without cheese, ½ cup	125
sticks, pieces ¾ to 2¾-inch long, ½ cup	95
Pumpkin (A), ½ cup	40
Sauerkraut, canned, ½ cup	20
Spinach (A,C), ½ cup	25
Squash	
summer, ½ cup	15
winter	
baked (A), mashed, ½ cup	65
boiled (A), mashed, ½ cup	45
Sweet Potatoes (A)	
baked in skin, 5 × 2-inch, one	160
candied, 2½-inches long, one-half	160
canned, mashed, ½ cup	140

Fruits (raw)	Calories
Apples, 2¾-inch-diameter, one	80
Apricots (A), 3 (about ¼ pound)	55
Avocados	
California varieties, 10 ounce, one-half	190
Florida varieties, 16 ounce, one-half	205
Bananas	
one 6- to 7-inch banana (about ⅓ pound)	85
one 8- to 9-inch banana (about ⅖ pound)	100
Berries	
blackberries, ½ cup	40
blueberries, ½ cup	45
raspberries	
black, ½ cup	50
red, ½ cup	35
strawberries (CC), ½ cup	30
Cantaloupe (A,CC), 5-inch melon, one-half	80
Cherries	
sour, ½ cup	30
sweet, ½ cup	40
Dates, "fresh" and dried, pitted, cut, ½ cup	245
Figs	
fresh, 3 small	95
dried, 1 large	60
Grapefruit (CC)	
white, half of a 3¾-inch fruit	45
sections, ½ cup	40
pink or red, half of 3¾-inch fruit	50
Grapes	
slip skin (Concord, Delaware, Niagara, etc.),	
½ cup	35
adherent skin (Malaga, Thompson seedless,	
Flame Tokay, etc.), ½ cup	55
Honeydew melon (C), 2 × 7-inch wedge	50
Oranges (CC), 2 ⅝-inch, one	65
Peaches	
slices, ½ cup	30
whole, 2½-inch peach (about ¼ pound)	40
Pears, 3½ × 2½ inch, one	100
Pineapple, diced, ½ cup	40
Plums	
damson, 1 inch (2 ounces), five	35
Japanese, 2⅛-inch (about 2½ ounces), one	30
Tangerines (C), 2⅜-inch tangerine (about ¼	
pound), one	40
Watermelon (C), one 2-pound wedge	110